EBP
This product is evidence based

Evidence-Based Competency Management *for the* Intensive Care Unit

SECOND EDITION

hcPro

Evidence-Based Competency Management for the Intensive Care Unit, Second Edition, is published by HCPro, Inc.

 5 4 3 2 1

First edition published 2004. Second edition published 2008.

ISBN 978-1-60146-153-7

HCPro, Inc., provides information resources for the healthcare industry.

HCPro, Inc., is not affiliated in any way with The Joint Commission, which owns the JCAHO and Joint Commission trademarks.

MAGNET™, MAGNET RECOGNITION PROGRAM®, and ANCC MAGNET RECOGNITION® are trademarks of the American Nurses Credentialing Center (ANCC). The products and services of HCPro, Inc. and The Greeley Company are neither sponsored nor endorsed by the ANCC.

Barbara A Brunt, MA, MN, RN-BC, Author
Adrianne E. Avillion, DEd, RN, Contributing Author
Gwen A. Valois, MS, RN, BC, Contributing Author
Jane G. Alberico, MS, RN, CEN, Contributing Author
Emily Sheahan, Group Publisher
Rebecca Hendren, Senior Managing Editor
Lindsey Cardarelli, Associate Editor
Audrey Doyle, Copyeditor
Janell Lukac, Layout Artist
Patrick Campagnone, Cover Designer
Liza Banks, Proofreader
Darren Kelly, Books Production Supervisor
Susan Darbyshire, Art Director
Claire Cloutier, Production Manager
Jean St. Pierre, Director of Operations

Advice given is general. Readers should consult professional counsel for specific legal, ethical, or clinical questions. Arrangements can be made for quantity discounts. For more information, contact:

HCPro, Inc.
P.O. Box 1168
Marblehead, MA 01945
Telephone: 800/650-6787 or 781/639-1872
Fax: 781/639-2982
E-mail: *customerservice@hcpro.com*

Visit HCPro at its World Wide Web sites:
www.hcpro.com* and *www.hcmarketplace.com

4/2008
21415

Contents

List of figures

About the author

Barbara A. Brunt, MA, MN, RN-BC

Barbara A. Brunt, MA, MN, RN-BC, is Director of Nursing Education and Staff Development for Summa Health System in Akron, OH. She has held a variety of staff development position, including educator, coordinator, and director for the past 30 years. Brunt has presented on a variety of topics both locally and nationally, and has published numerous articles, chapters in books, and books. She served as a section editor for all three editions of the *Core Curriculum for Staff Development* published by the National Nursing Staff Development Organization (NNSDO) and coauthored a book *Nursing Professional Development: Nursing Review and Resource Manual*, published by the American Nurses Credentialing Center Institute for Credentialing Innovation. She was the author of *Competencies for Staff Educators: Tools to Evaluate and Enhance Nursing Professional Development*, published by HCPro, Inc.

Brunt holds a master's degree in community health education from Kent State University and a master's degree in nursing from the University of Dundee in Scotland. Her research has focused on competencies. Brunt maintains certification in Nursing Professional Development and has been active in numerous professional associations. She is currently serving a two-year term as President of NNSDO, and a term as second vice-president for the Delta Omega Chapter of Sigma Theta Tau International. She has received awards for excellence in writing, nursing research, leadership, and staff development.

About the contributing authors

Adrianne E. Avillion, DEd, RN

Adrianne E. Avillion, DEd, RN, is the owner of Avillion's Curriculum Design in York, PA. She specializes in designing continuing education programs for healthcare professionals and freelance medical writing. She also offers consulting services in work redesign, quality improvement, and staff development.

Avillion has published extensively, including serving as editor of the first and second editions of *The Core Curriculum for Staff Development*. Her most recent publications include *Evidence-Based Staff Development: Strategies to Create, Measure, and Refine Your Program, A Practical Guide to Staff Development: Tools and Techniques for Effective Education,* and *Designing Nursing Orientation: Evidence-Based Strategies for Effective Programs*, all published by HCPro, Inc. in Marblehead, MA, and *Nurse Entrepreneurship: The Art of Running Your Own Business*, published by Creative Health Care Management in Minneapolis, MN. She is also a frequent presenter at conferences and conventions devoted to the specialty of continuing education and staff development.

Gwen A. Valois, MS, RN, BC

Gwen A. Valois, MS, RN, BC, is the director of organizational development at Medical City Dallas Hospital in Dallas. She has clinical expertise in pediatrics and has served for more than 25 years in various clinical educational and leadership roles.

Valois received her BSN from Texas Woman's University, her master's degree in human resource management and development from National Louis University, and holds certification from the American Nurses Credentialing Center in nursing professional development.

Jane G. Alberico, MS, RN, CEN

Jane G. Alberico, MS, RN, CEN, has more than 30 years of nursing practice in healthcare. She received her bachelor's of science degree from the University of Kentucky and master's degree in health science instruction, with a minor in healthcare administration, from Texas Woman's University.

Alberico is a certified emergency nurse whose clinical expertise includes medical-surgical, home health, pain management, and emergency care. She has served in faculty and leadership roles in school and hospital settings. She is a national speaker for various topics and is currently the supervisor for clinical education at Medical City Dallas Hospital in Dallas.

Preface

Before you use any methodology for validating and assessing the competency of your nurses to deliver safe patient care, it is essential that you have a system in place for verifying that your nurses are who they say they are prior to allowing them on your units.

This might sound obvious, but stories of nurses faking credentials, hopping from job to job in various states, and harming patients are stark reminders that you must be diligent in verifying any nursing applicant's licensure, criminal background, education, and employment history.

Nurse-credentialing processes at some facilities may be inadequate. Nurses who have had action taken against them by another state nursing board, have a criminal history, or have incomplete education may slip by and end up working in direct contact with your patients, making those patients vulnerable and your facility liable. You should examine your organization's policies to make sure they protect your patients, and sufficiently screen applicants for dangerous nurses or imposters.

Credentialing nurses falls to the HR department in most facilities, and the medical staff office handles physician and advance-practice RN credentialing. For advice on credentialing nurses, HR administrators can consult their colleagues in the medical staff office, who most likely already have an established credentialing process in place.

Here are some steps you can take to verify nurses' credentials and to ensure your patients' safety and your facility's integrity.

Step 1: Gather applicant information

The application for employment should be thorough and should obtain the information needed to ensure patient safety in your facility. Ask for the following:

- The applicant's name and any other names he or she has used (e.g., a maiden name)
- Education, the degree obtained, and the name and location of the educational institution
- Professional licensure, the state in which the license was issued, the date issued, the license number, and the expiration date
- Disciplinary actions on the license
- Specialty certification
- Employment history

With many new nursing schools starting up, the organization needs to determine whether it requires nursing applicants to be graduates of an accredited school of nursing. New programs cannot apply for National League for Nursing Accreditation Commission accreditation until after their first class has graduated, which means that organizations that require graduation from an accredited school cannot hire any graduates of these programs.

That also requires that the accreditation status of all schools from which a potential applicant graduated must be verified prior to hire. Is licensure to practice as a nurse in that state sufficient? Whatever policy the organization decides to follow must be followed consistently, and must be reflected in the job descriptions.

It is also important to determine whether the applicant has even been convicted or pleaded guilty or no contest to the following:

- Criminal charges (other than speeding violations)
- Drug- or alcohol-related offenses

If either one of these situations applies, ask the applicant to specify the charges and the dates on which they occurred. Finally, inquire whether he or she has ever been suspended, sanctioned, or otherwise restricted from participating in any private, federal, or state health insurance program (e.g., Medicare or Medicaid) or similar federal, state, or health agency.

Step 2: Verify the applicant's information

Verify to the best of your ability the information you obtained on the application. Even if you don't find anything, document each verification step to further reduce your hospital's liability.

Some facilities hire a third party to verify this information, but most often the HR department performs this task. Either way, make sure a specific, established process is in place.

The best method of checking an applicant's qualifications is to use primary source verification, including education, licensure, and past employment. For the most accurate and up-to-date information, you should check the state board in every state that the applicant nurse has worked. Most state licensing boards post licensure information on their Web sites.

Many organizations require criminal background checks on all applicants, even if the state nursing board runs checks on its own. Nurses may have committed a crime after receiving their licenses. In most states, the responsibility is on nurses to notify the state board it they are convicted of a crime, but they may or may not do so, which puts your facility at risk.

Another important part of the process is to check federal sanctions lists. If you hire a nurse who has been sanctioned by the Office of Inspector General or General Services Administration, you could be fined thousands of dollars. Reasons for sanctions include everything from defaulting on student loans to Medicare fraud.

Here are some other potential "red flags" to consider:

- **Gaps in job history:** HR professionals are well aware of this red flag, but be sure to ask about the gaps. Understand that there could be a perfectly good explanation, such as the birth of a child or a family emergency.

- **Moving from state to state:** When an applicant moves around a lot, his or her licensure information could be buried or lost. Therefore, be sure to check the status of the license in each state in which the applicant practiced.

- **Job hopping:** HR professionals are well aware of this pattern as well, and they will look twice at any applicant with evidence of it. But be sure to call each employer and verify that no disciplinary actions were taken against the applicant.

Step 3: Continually verify the employee's license after the hire date

Most facilities check nurses' licenses when they are up for renewal to make sure they are current and active. However, it is crucial that you institute a process to verify licensure status more often as well.

Ensure that your policy spells out that it is the nurse's responsibility to report any disciplinary action taken against his or her license over the course of his or her employment. If your nurses do not report such action, they could be working on your unit with a suspended or inactive license and you would have no idea. Many boards of nursing post disciplinary actions against nurses in that state, which can be used as another method to ensure that all employees have a current license with no restriction.

Creating a new credential-verification process or updating your current process is a very important prerequisite to the competency assessment process.

How to use this book

Evidence-Based Competency Management for the Intensive Care Unit, Second Edition will help you understand the basics of competency validation and assessment and discuss the steps you need to take to develop a process for performing these assessments at your organization.

In addition, this book provides you with evidence-based sample tools that will help get you started.

The appendix contains 49 evidence-based sample competency validation skill sheets. The skill sheets are organized into two sections: General and Intensive Care Unit. In addition, the appendix contains 24 role-related checklists, which can be used for orientation, training, or review purposes. The first page of each section contains a table of contents, which lists the name and page number of each skill sheet included in that section.

All of the content in the skill sheets was contributed or updated by Summa Health System Hospitals in Akron, OH. This content has been reprinted with the permission of this organization.

Customizable, electronic versions of all the skill sheets can be found on the CD-ROM accompanying the book. We have also included a copy of the "Competencies Analyzer" on your CD-ROM. This easy-to-use spreadsheet will help your unit or department managers organize their competency assessment program.
A complete list of tools included on the CD-ROM can be found in the "How to use the CD-ROM section."

Putting your skill sheets to work

The template used to standardize the appearance of these skills sheets appears on your CD-ROM. Save this blank template to your computer and use it to create additional skill sheets for your organization.

Duplicate this blank sheet as many times as needed. Type in content as you would into any table created using Microsoft's word-processing software to customize the sheets to fit your organization's needs, using the information discussed in this manual.

Here is a quick look at one of the skill sheets:

Name, date, skill – the section includes a space for the name of the employee whose competency is being validated, the date the validation is taking place, and the name of the skill being validated. Consider adding a second identifier, such as the employee number, to this section.

We have already provided the name of the skills for each of the skill sheets included in the manual. As we discuss in Chapter 2, however, all the competencies validated by your organization will not be technical or skill-based competencies, such as using a blood-glucose meter. Therefore, when customizing these sheets for validation on an interpersonal competency or a cultural competency, consider changing the term "skill" to "behavior" as a more accurate way to incorporate the elected required of these competencies.

Steps, completed, comments – This section is set up in a typical checklist format. After each step is successfully completed, the validator would add a check to the "completed" column. Consider changing the term "steps" to "performance criteria" when creating sheets for competencies that may not conform to a step-by-step format. The validator can use the "comments" column to record statements such as "needs reinforcement for steps" or "reteaching required."

Self-assessment – The validator should ask the employee to do a self-assessment of his or her competence on the skill being validated. Use this section to check off the appropriate response.

Evaluation/validation methods – This box contains some of the more common methodologies used to validate competencies. The validator should note which method was used in association with the skill sheet to validate the competency.

Levels – Consideration for the level of proficiency should be made when validating competencies (refer to Chapter 2). The level of proficiency (i.e., beginner, intermediate, expert) should coincide with the experience level of the employee. Should the level not coincide, then remediation should be planned to achieve the desired level of competence.

Type of validation – In this section, the validator can specify whether this competency validation tool was used during orientation, during an annual competency assessment, or at another point during the competency validation process.

Employee observer signature – Have both the employee and the validator (i.e., observer) sign the completed tool. This helps ensure the employee was an active participant in the process and that he or she understands and acknowledges this piece of the competency validation process.

How to use the files on your CD-ROM

The following file names correspond with figures listed in the book, *Evidence-Based Competency Management for the Intensive Care Unit, Second Edition*

sstemp.rtf	Blank skillsheet template
analyze.xls	Competencies Analyzer
Fig3-1.rtf	Figure 3.1: Essential functions
Fig4-1.rtf	Figure 4.1: Successful completion of competency assessment training form
Fig5-1.rtf	Figure 5.1: New competency assessment checklist
Fig6-2.rtf	Figure 6.2: Competency-based orientation checklist
Fig6-3.rtf	Figure 6.3: Nursing assistant orientation checklist

General:

General1.rtf	ABG Interpretation
General2.rtf	Annual Competency Performance—Quality of Instruction
General3.rtf	Arjo Ceiling Lift
General4.rtf	Assessment/Validation of Competencies
General5.rtf	Assisting Adult with Feeding
General6.rtf	Blood Glucose Meter
General7.rtf	Blood Pressure Measurement – Automatic
General8.rtf	Blood Pressure Measurement – Manual
General9.rtf	Digital Holter Hookup (Diagnostic Cardiology)
General10.rtf	Emergency Preparedness
General11.rtf	Falls Prevention (Get Up and Go)
General12.rtf	Fit Testing for N-95 Respirator Mask
General13.rtf	Intake and Output
General14.rtf	Medication Administration
General15.rtf	Oxygen Administration
General16.rtf	Presentation Skills
General17.rtf	Regulating and Monitoring IV Rate
General18.rtf	Service Excellence
General19.rtf	Thrombolytic Therapy
General20.rtf	Thrombus, Chronic versus Acute
General21.rtf	Use of Automated External Defibrillator (Heartstream FR2)
General22.rtf	Venipuncture with Winged Needle

Intensive Care Unit:

Icu1.rtf Arterial Duplex Graft
Icu2.rtf Arterial Line Monitoring
Icu3.rtf Barthel and Rankin Scores
Icu4.rtf Bipolar ECG Identification – Cardiac Rehab
Icu5.rtf Camino Intracranial Pressure Monitoring
Icu6.rtf Code Management – Critical Care
Icu7.rtf Codman External Drainage System II
Icu8.rtf Dialysis Fistula Duplex
Icu9.rtf Discontinuing Esophagogastric Tamponade Tube
Icu10.rtf Echocardiogram – Cardiology
Icu11.rtf Electroencephalogram (EEG) – Routine
Icu12.rtf Excel Care ES Bariatric Bed
Icu13.rtf Femostop Application
Icu14.rtf Hemaquet Removal Post Catheterization
Icu15.rtf Identification of Pseudoaneurysm
Icu16.rtf Lead Placement for Stress Testing
Icu17.rtf Mechanical Ventilation
Icu18.rtf Medtronic Pulse Generator
Icu19.rtf Miami J Cervical Collar
Icu20.rtf Nasopharyngeal/Tracheal Suctioning
Icu21.rtf Neurological Exam
Icu22.rtf Preparing for Intubation
Icu23.rtf Pulmonary Artery Pressure Catheter
Icu24.rtf Spinal Cord Monitoring
Icu25.rtf Thrombolytic Therapy
Icu26.rtf Ventricular Drain
Icu27.rtf Versacare Bed

Role Related:

Role1.rtf Acid Mixing
Role2.rtf Adding Toner to Fax
Role3.rtf Administrative Associate Accurate Charging
Role4.rtf Appointment Scheduling – Diabetes Center
Role5.rtf Age-Specific Competency Checklist RN/LPN
Role6.rtf Age-Specific Competency Checklist SA/AA
Role7.rtf Behavioral Health Associate Skills Assessment/Evaluation
Role8.rtf Bicarb Mixing
Role9.rtf Charge Entry
Role10.rtf Charge Nurse Assessment/Evaluation
Role11.rtf Defibrillator Function — Daily Check (Lifepak 9)
Role12.rtf Discharge Bed/Bassinette Cleaning for Environmental Associates
Role13.rtf Hospital Outpatient Profile (HOP) Charges
Role14.rtf Insurance Precertification Authorization

Role15.rtf	LPN Skills Assessment/Evaluation
Role16.rtf	Nursing Assistant Orientation Skills Assessment/Evaluation
Role17.rtf	Nursing Student Technician Competency Checklist
Role18.rtf	Private Duty RN/LPN Competency Evaluation
Role19.rtf	Registration
Role20.rtf	RN Skills Assessment/Evaluation
Role21.rtf	Sitter Guidelines
Role22.rtf	Telephone Skills
Role23.rtf	Telephone Skills (Problem Solving)
Role24.rtf	Unit Secretary Skills Assessment/Evaluation

To adapt any of the files to your own facility, simply follow the instructions below to open the CD.

If you have trouble reading the forms, click on "View," and then "Normal." To adapt the forms, save them first to your own hard drive or disk (by clicking "File," then "Save as," and changing the system to your own). Then change the information to fit your facility, and add or delete any items that you wish to change. Installation instructions

This product was designed for the Windows operating system and includes Word files that will run under Windows 95/98 or greater. The CD will work on all PCs and most Macintosh systems. To run the files on the CD/ROM, take the following steps:

1. Insert the CD into your CD/ROM drive.
2. Double-click on the "My Computer" icon, next double-click on the CD drive icon.
3. Double-click on the files you wish to open.
4. Adapt the files by moving the cursor over the areas you wish to change, highlighting them, and typing in the new information using Microsoft Word.
5. To save a file to your facility's system, click on "File" and then click on "Save As." Select the location where you wish to save the file and then click on "Save."
6. To print a document, click on "File" and then click on "Print."

Introduction

The focus on competence and evidence-based practice (EBP) is pervasive in healthcare today. Not only do the various regulatory agencies require assessment and documentation of competence of staff members, but the expectation is that organizations use evidence-based practice to provide quality care.

EBP is the process of making clinical decisions based on the most current and valid research and high-quality data available, with the goal of improving patient safety and decreasing the number of medical errors (Avillion 2007).

The second edition of this book includes the evidence for all the competencies that are provided. It should not be assumed that the competencies in the first edition were not based on current literature or evidence, but that information was not included on the competency itself. In this edition, the evidence base for each competency is included as part of the competency itself.

For the second edition, information in all the chapters has been updated to provide current resources on the competency management process. Chapter 1 outlines why competency validation is required, Chapter 2 defines competency validation, and Chapter 3 discusses including information on why competency validation should be a part of job descriptions and the performance-evaluation process. Chapter 4 focuses on the training needed for staff to perform competency validation, and Chapter 5 provides suggestions on keeping up with new competencies. How to use the skills checklists is described in Chapter 6.

There are 73 competency validation skills sheets included in this edition. Some of the skills in the first edition were deleted and others were added based on current practice and best evidence. In addition to the categories included in the first edition, there is another category added for general checklists that are role-related. These bonus checklists focus on specific skills required of various care providers, so these do not include references. The checklists can be adapted for the specific needs of your organization.

I hope you find the information in this second edition helpful whether you are developing a competency management program or refining ones you currently have in place.

REFERENCES

1. Avillion, Adrianne E. (2007). *Evidence-Based Staff Development: Strategies to Create, Measure, and Refine Your Program.* Marblehead, MA: HCPro, Inc.

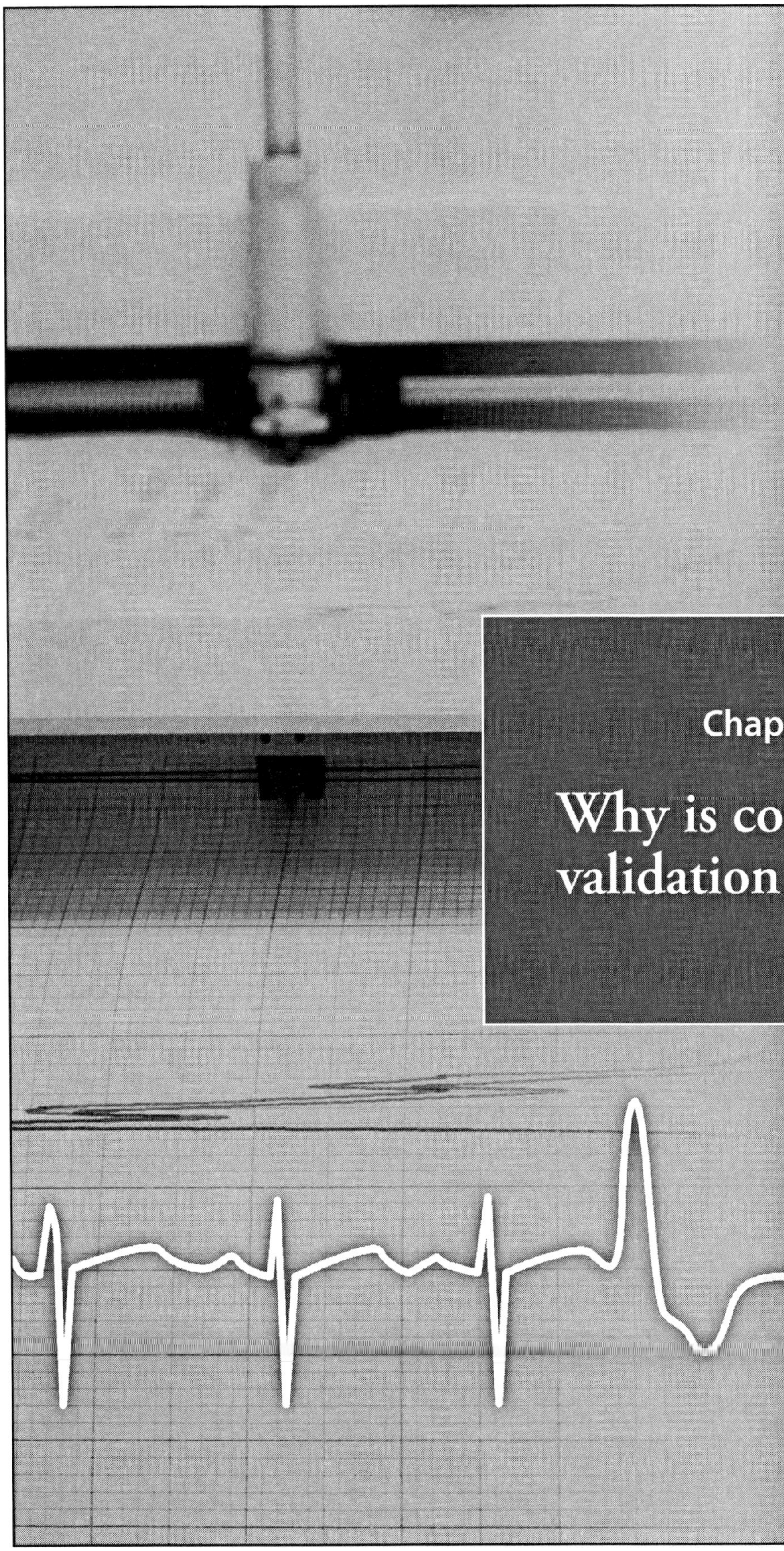

Chapter 1

Why is competency validation required?

Chapter 1

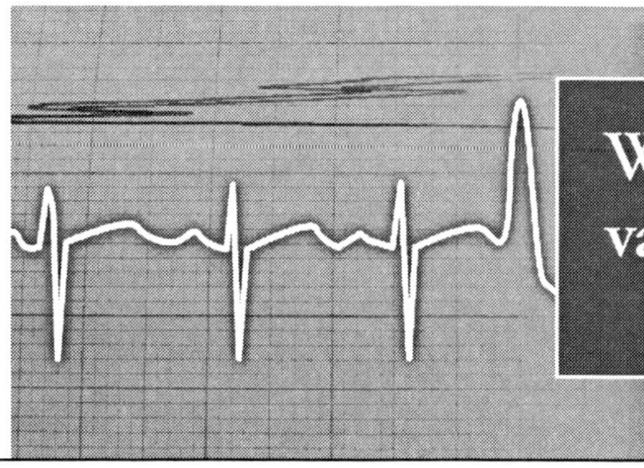

Why is competency validation required?

Learning objectives

After reading this chapter, the participant should be able to:

- Design a competency plan to effectively assess employee competence

Regulating competence

Does it seem as though regulatory survey teams visit you every day? Sometimes the survey is announced and sometimes it's a surprise, but every time, the surveyors—regardless of whom they represent—are concerned about "competency."

The definition of this word is in the eye of the beholder. *Webster's New World College Dictionary*, for instance, defines *competent* as "well qualified, capable, fit" (Agnes 2006). The American Nurses Association (ANA) defines *competency* as "an expected level of performance that results from an integration of knowledge, skills, abilities, and judgment" (ANA 2007). In healthcare, however, it's not so simple. Your healthcare staff make decisions and carry out responsibilities and job duties that affect patients' lives. When the goal is to achieve positive patient outcomes—whether to cure or manage a chronic disease process, or to allow someone to die a dignified death—will "sufficient ability" be good enough? Should competency apply only to clinical bedside nursing? Should an RN case manager have to meet the same competency requirements as a critical-care staff nurse? No, no, and no.

Evidence-based practice involves supporting your actions with research and data, and basing competencies in evidence is becoming the standard in competency validation. Researchers have identified best practices for patient care based on evidence, so when assessing staff members' competence, they should be assessed based on their provision of evidence-based care. By instituting evidence-based practice in your competency assessment, you ensure the methods by which you are validating your staff members' skills are established and grounded in research. In this book, you are provided with references to the original research so you are able to institute evidence-based competency assessment at your facility.

Protecting the public

Regulatory agencies are rampant in the healthcare industry. Their purpose is to protect the public and to ensure a consistent standard of care for patients and families. Initially, there was only the Joint Commission on Accreditation of Hospitals (JCAH). Ernest Codman, a physician, proposed the standardization process for hospitals in 1910, and the American College of Surgeons developed the Minimum Standards for Hospitals in 1917 and officially transferred its program to the JCAH in 1952. A trickling of new agencies followed, and in 1964, the JCAH started charging for surveys. JCAH changed its name to the Joint Commission on Accreditation of Healthcare Organizations (JCAHO) in 1987 and is now known simply as The Joint Commission (The Joint Commission 2007).

The list of regulators today now looks like an alphabet soup. Political debates regarding the effectiveness of these agencies have multiplied in recent years. In July 2004, for example, the Centers for Medicare & Medicaid Services (CMS) began to criticize the validity of Joint Commission accreditations. However, since its inception, The Joint Commission has never had federal oversight (Knight 2004). In some cases, criteria for federally mandated CMS regulatory standards may exceed those of The Joint Commission.

For acute-care facilities, the agencies that "oversee" patient care and thus require competency assessment may now include the following:

- The Joint Commission
- CMS
- National Quality Foundation
- The Leapfrog Group

- State departments of health and human services
- State medical foundations
- ANA
- State Board of Nurse Examiners (BNE)
- Health Quality Improvement Initiatives
- Occupational Safety & Health Administration (OSHA)
- College of American Pathologists (CAP)
- Office of Inspector General
- Quality improvement organizations
- Agency for Healthcare Research and Quality
- The U.S. Food and Drug Administration
- Centers for Disease Control and Prevention (CDC)

Add to this a list of your hospital's competency assessment initiatives. Most of these initiatives revolve around the mission, vision, and value statements for the organization. Indicators may include:

- Patient satisfaction
- Physician satisfaction
- Employee health and pride
- Fiscal responsibility
- Community involvement
- Risk management

Those of us working in healthcare started our careers wanting to improve human life, and it is frustrating at times when it seems that the bureaucracy of regulatory mandates keeps growing. But the business of healthcare must consist of personnel who are both caring and able to perform their jobs safely and correctly. Remember that the provision of quality care and services depends on knowledgeable, competent healthcare providers. Every organization should have a competency plan in place to ensure that performance expectations based on job-specific position descriptions are consistently met.

You must design your competency plan with consideration given to:

- The mission, vision, and values of your organization
- The needs of patients and families served
- The extended community
- New services or technologies planned for future services
- Special needs required for particular healthcare situations
- Current standards of professional practice
- Applicable legal and regulatory agency requirements
- Organizational policies and procedures

In addition, the organization should foster learning on a continual basis. The CEO and nurse executive should mandate this learning environment and hold the leadership team and staff accountable for expected outcomes (Joint Commission Resources 2008). The entire organization must foster a work environment that helps employees discover what they need to learn for self-growth.

What's the return on this investment? A positive patient/family outcome. The outcome may be improved health, the ability to manage a chronic disorder, or even a dignified death.

A consistent process for competency assessment is essential throughout the organization for all job classes, contract personnel, and, when indicated, affiliating schools. There must be a centralized, organized approach that moves seamlessly throughout the continuum of care and ensures the same standard or practice for all of the patients and families it serves. If your main policies and procedures say one thing but certain departments or units develop their own policies and procedures that say something else, you are in trouble.

Generating tons of paperwork does not ensure competency in practice. Use the KISS method: "Keep it simple, smarty." Although documenting that standards are being met is important, regulatory surveyors are moving away from looking at paper. The trend is to interview patients, staff members, physicians, vendors, and members of the leadership team to see evidence of compliance. And now more than ever, there are expectations to move beyond merely verifying whether nurses are "competent." Thanks in part to advances in technology, nurses have been catapulted into more advanced and specialized care. Entire nursing divisions in hospital settings may now apply for American Nurses Credentialing Center (ANCC) Magnet Recognition Program® designation. Designations such as this and the Malcolm Baldrige National Quality Award are raising the bar for practice by empowering nurses to demand excellence in delivering care.

Instead of telling you months in advance the date on which it will arrive at your hospital, the regulatory agency may show up at your door at any time without advance notice. In fact, Joint Commission surveyors began doing so in 2006. Therefore, it is vital for you and your organization to be survey-ready every day. Ongoing performance must be measured and assessed. If individual members of your healthcare organization do not meet the standards you've established, individuals and the leadership team must develop a system for ongoing validation and assessment of personnel based on those standards. Remember: Competency assessment would be necessary even if it were not an accreditation standard.

It is worth framing this discussion on the expectations of regulatory agencies, because understanding their motivations and complying with their recommendations will result in a better understanding of what an effective competency assessment process should look like. What do these regulatory agencies want? In our upcoming discussion of The Joint Commission, we will also introduce the concepts of other state and federal agencies.

The Joint Commission

The Joint Commission is still considered to be the leader in healthcare accreditation. Standards devoted to competency are woven through The Joint Commission's accreditation manual, from the leadership chapter to the environment of care chapter. It uses elements of performance (EPs) to determine hospitals' compliance with standards. The Joint Commission's 2008 HR standards listed in the following section summarize its expectations for competency (Joint Commission Resources 2008).

Standard HR.1.20

A staff member's qualifications are consistent with his or her job responsibilities.

This requirement pertains to staff members, students, and volunteers who work in the same capacity as staff members who provide care, treatment, and services. This also includes contract staff members.

It seems simple enough, doesn't it? Steve Doe applies to be an emergency department (ED) staff RN. HR representatives compare what Steve Doe put on his application to the RN job description for an ED staff nurse to determine whether he meets the qualifications for the position. The criteria on the job description state, "Licensed RN in the state of Texas. Minimum of two years recent clinical experience in an ED required. Current card in basic life support for healthcare providers, advanced cardiac life support, and pediatric advanced life support required. Certified emergency nurse preferred." Steve Doe had better meet these requirements.

As we indicated in the Preface, the process for verifying these credentials is of utmost importance to the safety of your patients. Your organization needs a system to ensure that your nurses are who they say they are and have the experience and documentation to back it up. A surveyor may ask an ED nurse (who happens to be Steve Doe), "What is required to work in this department?" The nurse tells the surveyor what was required for his position. The surveyor may then ask for an ED staff RN job description as well as Steve's file to see whether the hospital did indeed verify that all the screening requirements were met and that there is a record indicating that the requirements are still being met.

Standard HR.2.10

The hospital provides initial orientation.

The EPs establish that this standard applies to each staff member, student, and volunteer at your facility. The EPs encompass the following:

- Key elements of orientation that must occur before staff members provide care
- Orientation of the staff to identified key elements prior to providing care
- The hospital's mission and goals

- Organization- and relevant unit-, setting-, or program-specific (e.g., safety and infection control) policies and procedures
- Specific job duties and responsibilities and unit-, setting-, or program-specific job duties related to safety and infection control
- Cultural diversity and sensitivity
- Patient rights and ethical aspects of care, treatment, and services and the process to address ethical issues

In addition, the forensic staff (i.e., police who bring in prisoners) must know how to:

- Interact with patients
- Respond to life safety codes
- Communicate through appropriate channels
- Define their roles in clinical seclusion and restraint

It is expected that, during orientation, the hospital assesses and documents the competency level of the new hire so that by the end of orientation the person is deemed competent (sample orientation competency assessment tools for an RN and nurse assistant appear in Chapter 6). This standard highlights the fact that competence in nursing is not a one-size-fits-all arrangement. Although your ability to synthesize your competency assessment practices across your entire organization will ultimately determine your success, you must be able to customize your tools and process to their intended audience. However, keep in mind that the organization is not expected to shoulder this responsibility alone. Provision 5.2 under the ANA's Code of Ethics states that the nurse "owes the same duties to self as to others, including the responsibility to preserve integrity and safety, to maintain competence, and to continue personal and professional growth" (ANA 2001).

As a result, state BNEs' rules and regulations may dictate competency expectations. These regulations vary, but many discuss competency pertaining to:

- Role delineation for "respondent superiors" (i.e., adult nurse practitioners, licensed practical nurses, licensed vocational nurses, new grads, and unlicensed personnel)
- Scopes of practice for patient care

- Peer review
- Informed consent
- Medication administration
- Pain management (including epidurals)
- Conscious sedation/analgesia
- Patient/family education
- Blood administration
- Population-specific care

Standard HR.2.20

Staff and licensed independent practitioners, as appropriate, can describe or demonstrate their roles and responsibilities relative to safety.

The EPs for this standard include:

- Risks within the hospital environment
- Actions to eliminate, minimize, and report risks
- Procedures to follow in the event of an adverse event
- Reporting processes for common problems, failures, and user errors

This standard coincides with the introduction of the National Patient Safety Goals (NPSGs) and new requirements by The Joint Commission. The NPSGs are derived from a sentinel event advisory group, and the requirements are generally more prescriptive than other Joint Commission requirements. They are based upon aggregate data following national trends of sentinel patient events. As of January 1, 2005, The Joint Commission began to incorporate NPSGs into the accreditation survey (Joint Commission 2007). The NPSGs highlight the link between competent patient care and safety. To fulfill your hospital's mission of delivering safe patient care, there is significant value in validating healthcare professionals' competencies associated with these goals.

Also note that licensed independent practitioners (LIPs) have been included in HR.2.20. An LIP is someone who is authorized by law and the hospital to "provide care and services without direction or supervision, within the scope of the individual's license and consistent with individually granted clinical privileges" (Joint Commission Resources 2008). LIPs give medical orders for patient care. The individual is credentialed through the hospital medical staff committee.

2008 National Patient Safety Goals

Goal #1. Improve the accuracy of patient identification.

- Use at least two patient identifiers when providing care, treatment, or services

Goal #2. Improve the effectiveness of communication among caregivers.

- For verbal or telephone orders or for telephonic reporting of critical test results, verify the complete order or test result by having the person receiving the information record and "read back" the complete order or test result
- Standardize a list of abbreviations, acronyms, symbols, and dose designations that are not to be used throughout the organization
- Measure and assess, and if appropriate, take action to improve the timeliness of reporting, and the timeliness of receipt by the responsible licensed caregiver, of critical tests and critical results and values
- Implement a standardized approach to "hand off" communications, including an opportunity to ask and respond to questions

Goal #3. Improve the safety of using medications.

Look-alike, sound-alike names for medications and concentrated electrolyte drug concentrations are sentinel events waiting to happen. Studies have been initiated regarding the advent of computer-based medication administration to improve the safety of such medications. For example, bar code scanning, the latest technological advance, may decrease medication errors. But with this new technology comes a new set of competencies. These competencies must be validated before care is initiated with the new technology, and your assessments must be ongoing. In addition, this goal expects you to:

- Identify and review at least annually look-alike, sound-alike drugs used in the organization
- Label all medications, medication containers (e.g., syringes, medicine cups, and basins) or other solutions on and off the sterile field
- Reduce the likelihood of patient harm associated with anticoagulation therapy

Goals #4–6. Not applicable.

Goal #7. Reduce the risk of healthcare-associated infections.

This includes:

- Compliance with World Health Organization or CDC hand hygiene guidelines
- Managing all cases of unanticipated death or loss of function from a healthcare-associated infection as a sentinel event

OSHA mandates competency in maintaining health requirements for those working in healthcare facilities. These OSHA competencies must be validated. Tuberculosis testing, use of personal protective equipment, use of needless systems, latex allergy requirements, and so on stress the need for those involved in direct patient care to be competent in delivering that care to your patients.

Goal #8. Accurately and completely reconcile medications across the continuum of care.

A process must be developed for obtaining and documenting a complete list of current patient medications—with the involvement of the patient—upon admission. The process includes a comparison of the medications the organization provides to those on the list. This list is communicated to the next provider of service upon transfer or referral within or outside of the organization and is provided to the patient on discharge from the organization. Goal #8 requires interpersonal communication and listening skills, competencies that are challenging but not impossible for your organization to validate.

Goal #9. Reduce the risk of patient harm resulting from falls.

For this goal, the organization must implement a fall reduction program, including an evaluation of the effectiveness of the program. Staff members, patients, and families must be educated on the fall reduction program.

Goals #10–12. Not applicable.

Goal #13. Encourage patients' active involvement in their own care as a patient safety strategy.
The organization must define and communicate the means for patients and their families to report concerns about safety and encourage them to do so. When patients know what to expect, they are more aware of possible errors and choices. Patients can be an important source of information regarding potential adverse events and hazardous conditions.

Goal #14. Not applicable.

Goal #15. The organization identifies safety risks inherent in its client population.

- The organization identifies clients at risk for suicide

Goal #16. Improve recognition and response to changes in a patient's condition. (Note: this requirement has a one-year phase-in period that includes defined expectations for planning, development, and testing ["milestones"] at three, six, and nine months in 2008, with the expectation of full implementation by January 1, 2009.)

- The organization selects a suitable method that enables healthcare staff members to directly request additional assistance from one or more specially trained individuals when the patient's condition appears to be worsening
- Formal education for urgent response policies and practices is conducted with the people who may request assistance and the people who may respond to those requests

Many organizations have implemented Rapid Response Teams to meet this standard. Early response to changes in a patient's condition may reduce cardiopulmonary arrests and patient mortality.

The list of NPSGs will probably lengthen with time. However, using evidence-based practice and benchmarking, facilities with the best-practice data to reduce risk and enhance patient safety will continue to drive competency in practice in the future.

Standard HR.2.30

Ongoing education, including inservices, training, and other activities, maintains and improves competence.

With this standard, The Joint Commission expects that measuring competency at your organization is an ongoing process. In other words, it isn't enough for you to assume that your system for validating competencies at orientation will cover your employees for the length of their employment. EPs for this standard expect:

- Training to occur when job responsibilities and duties change (e.g., when an ED nurse transfers to the neonatal ICU [NICU] but has never worked in a NICU setting).
- That participation in ongoing training will increase staff, student, or volunteer knowledge of work-related issues.
- Ongoing education to be appropriate to the needs of the population(s) served, safety, and infection prevention and control, and to comply with laws and regulations.
- Staff members to know how to manage and report unanticipated events.
- Inservices and staff education to incorporate methods of team training, when appropriate.
- That learning needs to be identified through performance improvement findings and other data analysis. Education is planned, implemented, and evaluated for effectiveness.
- Documentation of ongoing staff education.

Most state boards of nursing mandate continuing education requirements for nurses who apply for relicensure. Hospitals striving for recognition through the ANCC Magnet Recognition Program® are required to foster an environment of continual learning for their nursing staff or risk losing their designation. This standard underlines the need for ongoing education and competency validation at your organization.

Standard HR.3.10

Staff competence to perform job responsibilities is assessed, demonstrated, and maintained.

Once again, this standard stresses that competency assessment be an ongoing process. An EP for this standard may be point-of-care testing (POCT) for the CAP. For example, for CAP accreditation to be maintained, staff members must be competent to perform POCT (CAP Web site). This testing goes beyond knowing how to do a fingerstick test for blood-glucose testing. CAP wants to know who is allowed to do POCT. Are staff members involved in quality control testing and documentation as defined by hospital policy? What tests are allowed to be performed outside of the main hospital laboratory, and what areas are allowed to do what? Examples of POCT that may need to be validated include (but may not be limited to):

- Hemacult
- Urine dipstick
- Nitrazine pH
- Blood glucose

Competency and litigation

Regulatory agencies and legal issues are conjoined in HR.3.10. What is the link? Competency assessment is "systematic and allows for a measurable assessment of the person's ability to perform required activities" (Joint Commission Resources 2008). The EPs do not say that you have to use a certain form or have a certain methodology, but you do have to use a systematic measurable process.

In addition, whoever assesses competency must be qualified to do so. The leadership team must know the qualifications of the staff members caring for the patient population served and is accountable and responsible for maintaining a competent staff. For example, an ED nurse cannot deem another ED nurse competent in managing an overdose patient if the "assessor" has managed only one overdose patient. Peer review is critical to competency assessment, but careful consideration must be given to the process.

Plaintiffs' attorneys in legal cases use expert witnesses to verify issues related to competency. For example, the expert ED nurse called on the case of an overdose patient may manage several overdoses every day. This credible witness likely embodies the standard for excellence and competency in practice. If the patient had a negative outcome following a gastric lavage, the expert may be able to dispute the defendant organization's method used to measure competency of ED staff nurses caring for overdose patients.

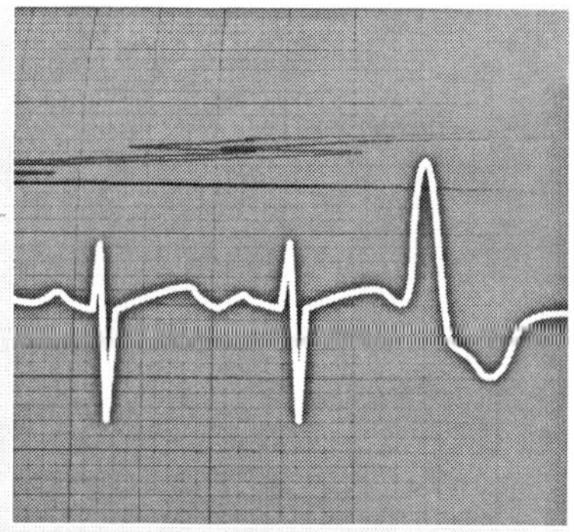

Case study

Surveyors tracing for competent care

The staff members at Healthcare Hospital are in their second day of a four-day Joint Commission survey. Wanda, the nurse surveyor, is in the critical-care unit (CCU) focusing on a tracer patient named Mrs. D., who was admitted from the ED. Mrs. D. tried to commit suicide in the ED. She was lavaged for her overdose, intubated, and transferred to the CCU.

The Joint Commission's tracer methodology strives to ensure that the same standard of care is used throughout the facility by retracing the care delivered to sample patients (or tracers), so Wanda asks the nurse manager to gather three caregivers associated with this patient's case. She also requests that she pull their personnel files because Wanda wants to first ask these nurses various questions regarding the care the patient received and their competency to deliver that care. Then she'll verify whether accreditation standards have been met by reviewing their files. The three employees are:

- A new graduate who is going through a critical-care internship
- An RN with 25 years of experience in critical care
- A certified nursing assistant (CNA) who is a foreign nurse preparing to sit for the boards in the United States

Wanda also wants to review the nurse manager's file to verify that she meets the competency standards required of her as a member of the leadership team at this facility; she wants to know what training she has had to become a leader. Wanda then proceeds to walk around the unit and delves further into the standards for hospital accreditation.

Based upon federal and state regulatory requirements discussed in this chapter, can you think of some of the important questions Wanda will ask the staff, physician, patient (if this vented patient can participate), and family?

Wanda may ask whether the new graduate is competent to take care of a ventilator patient. If so, how was that validated? If she is not competent, what is the action plan? If the nurse with 25 years of experience is her preceptor, how was she deemed competent? Can the CNA, who is a nurse in her country of origin, interpret the monitor strips correctly?

How would Wanda ensure the timely and accurate assessment of competencies for these personnel? Could she pull job descriptions? Performance evaluations? Competency checklists, or skill sheets? Is your organization ready for that?

Your organization must ask itself, "Are the right people taking care of the right patients for the right reasons?" Consider the following:

> **The decline of standards**
> A big-city school system requires a student in the seventh grade to be able to read as well as a fifth grader, who must be able to read as well as a fourth grader, who, in turn, must be able to read as well as a third grader. What's wrong with demanding that a seventh grader be required to read like a seventh grader? How would you like to be operated on by a brain surgeon who graduated from a school that allowed its students to be a year and a half behind in their skills?
> *—Author unknown*

REFERENCES

1. Agnes, M. (Ed). (2006). *Webster's New World College Dictionary*. Cleveland: Wiley Publishing.

2. ANA. (2001). *Code of Ethics for Nurses with Interpretive Statements*. Washington, DC: ANA.

3. ANA. (2007). *Position Statement on Competency*. Silver Springs, MD: ANA.

4. College of American Pathologists. (2007). Available at *www.cap.org*. Accessed November 25, 2007.

5. The Joint Commission. (2007). "A Journey Through the History of The Joint Commission." Available at *www.jointcommission.org/AboutUs/joint_commission_history.htm*. Accessed November 25, 2007.

6. Joint Commission Resources. (2008). *Comprehensive Accreditation Manual for Hospitals: The Official Handbook*. "GL-12." Oakbrook, IL: Joint Commission Resources.

7. Joint Commission Resources. (2008) *Comprehensive Accreditation Manual for Hospitals: The Official Handbook*. "HR2–HR13." Oakbrook, IL: Joint Commission Resources .

8. Joint Commission Resources. (2007). *Comprehensive Accreditation Manual for Hospitals: The Official Handbook*. "Standard NR3.10, *CAMH* Update 1, March 2007, p. NR-4." (Oakbrook, IL: Joint Commission Resources.

9. Joint Commission Resources. (2008). *Comprehensive Accreditation Manual for Hospitals: The Official Handbook*. "Standard NR3.10, *CAMH* Update 1, September 2006, p. HR-12." Oakbrook, IL: Joint Commission Resources.

10. Knight, Tom.(2004). "JCAHO Certification—Dissecting an Institution." *The Nurses' Lounge* September 2004: 26.

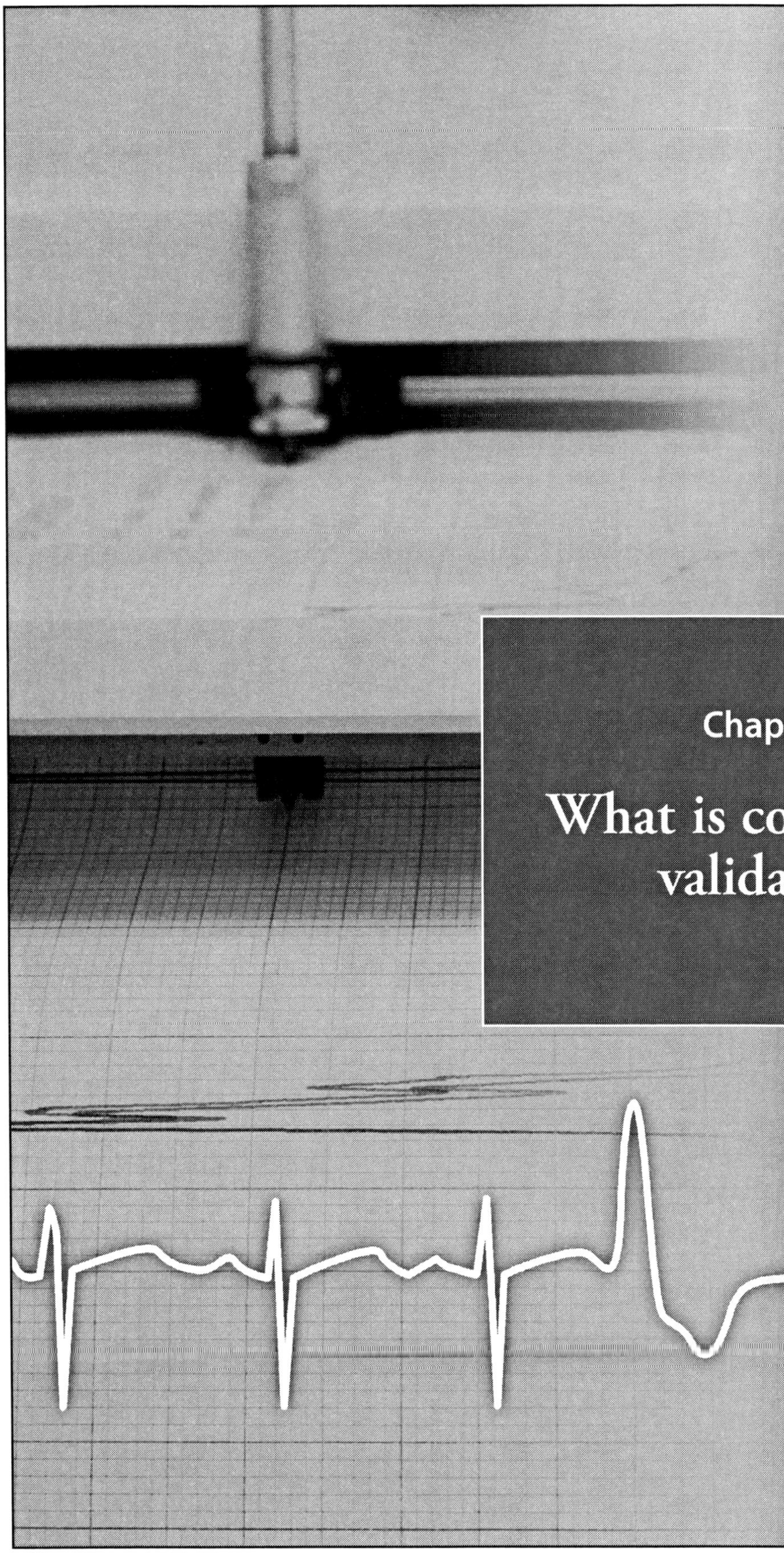

Chapter 2

What is competency validation?

Chapter 2

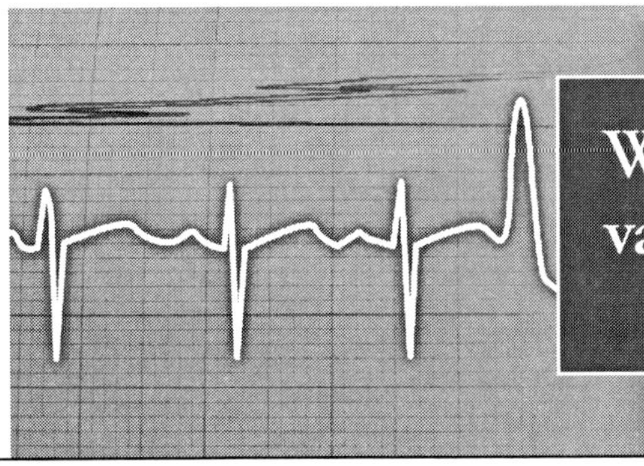

What is competency validation?

Learning objectives

After reading this chapter, the participant should be able to:

- Identify benefits of competency-based education
- Describe methods of validating competencies

Competency is an issue that affects nursing personnel in all practice settings. Increased pressure from multiple healthcare regulatory agencies and the public necessitates comprehensive evaluation of staff competency. The public demands that nurses demonstrate their competence. This chapter provides information on competency-based education (CBE), as well as on levels and domains of competency. Responsibility for competency validation and the difference between mandatory training and competencies are outlined. The chapter also describes methods for validating competence and options for mapping out or scheduling competencies.

Competency-based education

CBE is one approach commonly used to assess and validate competency. In many ways, CBE reflects a pragmatic concern for doing, not just knowing how to do. Competency models began to evolve during the 1960s as an approach to teacher education, and today CBE models are a widely applied approach to validating competence. In CBE, the learners' self-direction allows educators to act as facilitators to promote learners' goals and is compatible with adults' developmental needs.

Brunt identified that common characteristics of CBE include a learner-centered philosophy, real-life orientation, flexibility, clearly articulated standards, a focus on outcomes, and criterion-reference evaluation methods (Brunt 2007). Most CBE programs focus on outcomes rather than processes.

Generally, CBE programs focus on a specific role and setting and use criteria developed by expert practitioners. CBE emphasizes outcomes in terms of what individuals must know and be able to do and allows flexible pathways for achieving those outcomes. Figure 2.1 provides a comparison of CBE and traditional education.

Figure 2.1

Comparison of CBE and traditional education

Characteristic	CBE programs (Learner-centered)	Traditional education (Teacher-centered)
Basis of instruction	Student outcomes (competencies)	Specific information to be covered
Pace of instruction	Learner sets own pace in meeting objectives	All proceed at pace determined by instructor
How proceed from task to task	Master one task before moving to another	Fixed amount of time on each module
Focus of instruction	Specific tasks included in role	Information that may or may not be part of role
Method of evaluation	Evaluated according to predetermined standards	Relate achievement of learner to other learners

A competency-based approach offers many benefits. These include:

- Having clear guidelines for everyone involved in the process
- Encouraging teamwork
- Enhancing skills and knowledge
- Increasing staff retention
- Reducing staff anxiety
- Improving nursing performance
- Ensuring compliance with the Joint Commission standard that all members of the staff are competent to fulfill their assigned responsibilities

Figure 2.2 provides a sample policy for a competency-based program.

Figure 2.2

Sample competency-based program policy

SUMMA HEALTH SYSTEM HOSPITALS
AKRON CITY HOSPITAL
SAINT THOMAS HOSPITAL

POLICY: Competency Based Program
SECTION: VI
PAGE: 4

PATIENT CARE SERVICES
STAFF POLICY AND PROCEDURE SECTION

SUBJECT:

Summa Health System Hospitals has adopted a competency-based program to ensure that nursing staff are prepared to deliver quality patient care. Assessment of competency begins with orientation and continues throughout employment.

An evaluation of each nursing staff member's competency is conducted at defined intervals throughout the individual's association with the hospital. Performance appraisals may be used as a measure of ongoing competency of nursing employees. Nursing staff members have access to ongoing continuing education programs to enhance their competency.

DEFINITIONS:

Department of Patient Care Services Orientation: Consists of centralized orientation and unit orientation. Some areas also have a divisional orientation.

- **Centralized Orientation:** Refers to the introduction, reinforcement, and demonstration of general required competencies that a nursing staff member needs to practice within any division of Summa Health System.
- **Divisional Orientation:** Refers to the introduction and application of general practice concepts related to the division assigned. Divisional orientation is reserved for specialties such as critical care, medical-surgical, and operating room.
- **Unit Orientation:** Refers to the clinical application of general and unit-specific competencies for a nursing staff member to practice on his/her assigned unit specialty, or patient population. It also includes geographic and social orientation.

Figure 2.2

Sample competency-based program policy (cont.)

Competency: Skill/activity identified by unit/ division that must be successfully performed to promote quality patient care. Competency is concerned with what the individual can do in the provision of patient care.

- **Departmental Competencies:** Competencies required for all staff assigned to direct patient care, such as BLS.
- **Divisional Competencies:** Selected competencies required within a specific nursing division or specialty, generally included in a curriculum specific to the division, or specialty, such as but not limited to,

  Obstetrics
  - Neonatal resuscitation

  Critical care
  - ACLS
  - EKG interpretation

  Behavioral health
  - Nonviolent crisis intervention

- **Unit-Competencies:** Unit-specific competencies required for nursing staff members working on that unit/specialty patient population.

Competence Assessment Process

Competence assessment for nursing staff and volunteers who are providing direct patient care is based on the following:

1. Populations served, including age ranges and specialties.
2. Competencies required for role and provision of care.
3. Competencies assessed during orientation.

Figure 2.2

Sample competency-based program policy (cont.)

4. Unit specific competencies that need to be assessed or reassessed on a yearly basis, based on care modalities, age ranges, techniques, procedures, technology, equipment, skills needed, or changes in law and regulations.

5. Appropriate assessment methods for the skill being assessed.

6. Delineation of who is qualified to assess competence.

7. Description of action taken when improvement activities lead to a determination that a staff member with performance problems is unable or unwilling to improve.

Ongoing Competence: Refers to periodic assessment of selected competencies for the nursing staff member practicing within a division and on a specific nursing unit; may be centralized or division/unit specific.

Required competency will include:

1. Annual performance appraisal.

2. Completion of mandatory organizational education and other inservices designated as mandatory for personnel.

3. BLS health care provider course or renewal every 2 years (RNs, LPNs, technicians, medical assistants).

4. BLS heartsaver course every 2 years (nursing assistants, unit secretaries).

5. Unit competencies.

Required specialty competencies will include the above as well as unit competencies. Each year unit based competencies will be reviewed by the unit manager and required competencies changed based on individual needs of the unit, identified QI needs or problems identified, changes in patient population, care modalities, technol-

Figure 2.2

Sample competency-based program policy (cont.)

ogy, etc. A complete list of chosen unit based competencies will be maintained in staff development.

DIVISIONAL COMPETENCIES (continued):

Assessing Competence

1. Competency checklists will be used to assess demonstrated and ongoing competence. This ensures consistency in evaluating the steps to perform the skill.

2. When introducing new technology or procedures into the clinical area, the initial training is done by individuals with documented experience in that procedure (e.g., physician, nurses from that specialty, vendor representatives, etc.). A core group of staff members or a single individual is trained and confirms competency of other staff members after they personally demonstrate competence in that skill.

3. Ongoing competence will be assessed by an individual with documented competence in that skill. That competence may be determined by their role (e.g., advanced practice nurse, staff development instructor, unit manager, specialty coordinator, etc.), frequency performing the skill, or by already having demonstrated competence in that skill.

Documentation of Competence

1. Each unit will have a Continuing Education Record and Employee Profile binder.

2. Each employee will have an individual record in the binder.

3. It is the responsibility of the individual staff member to complete the education record and employee profile.

4. Preceptors, Unit Managers and Associate Unit Managers can sign employees off on their competencies.

Figure 2.2

Sample competency-based program policy (cont.)

5. Approved list of preceptors by unit will be listed in the front of the binder.

6. All competency checklists specific to each department and division will be located in the front of the education binder.

7. The required competencies are listed on the Continuing Education Record and Employee Profile for department and division.

8. The staff required to complete the competency, activity, or self-learning packets are listed on the profile.

9. RNs are required to complete all competencies, activities or self-learning packets.

10. Competencies are to be completed by December of each year and will be utilized in annual performance appraisal.

11. Once the employee demonstrates competency to preceptor they need to have preceptor sign off on the employee profile.

12. Employees can fax or give this profile to education department to include information on electronic continuing education record (employee needs to submit copy of contact hour certificate).

13. The back of the profile is for staff document continuing education/contact hours, presentations that they have attended.

14. Employees still needed to sign their names that they completed the self-learning packet on sign in sheets.

15. Staff not able to accurately perform any competency will be referred to the Unit Manager. They will be given 30 days to meet this competency and will not be assigned to a patient who requires that competency during that

Figure 2.2

Sample competency-based program policy (cont.)

period. At the end of 30 days if they cannot meet the required competency they will be transferred from that area and reassigned to another area with an open position in which they meet the competencies. Continued failure to demonstrate required competencies leads to a practice plan for improvement and eventual termination.

REFERENCE:

Brunt, B. A. (2007). *Competencies for Staff Educators: Tools to Evaluate and Enhance Nursing Professional Development.* Marblehead, MA: HCPro

____

Mary H. Ward, BSN, MBA, RN, CNAA-BC
Vice President/CNO Patient Care Services

____

Barbara Brunt, MA, MN, RN-BC
Director, Nursing Education and
Staff Development

Source: Summa Health Systems Hospitals, Akron, OH. Reprinted with permission.

Defining competencies

Confusion surrounding the competency movement is a result of the numerous definitions used to address this concept, and definitions vary widely. The definition used in this chapter is that *competency* is a broad statement describing an aspect of practice that must be developed and demonstrated, and *competence* is the achievement and integration of many competencies into practice, or the overall ability to perform. Competency is about what people can do. It is the integration of cognitive, affective, and psychomotor domains of practice. It involves both the ability to perform in a given context and the capacity to transfer knowledge and skills to new tasks and situations.

Classifying competencies by domains and levels

Once an institution has a clear definition of competency, the next step is to classify competencies by domains and levels.

Domains of competency

Dorothy del Bueno, a recognized expert in nursing CBE, described three domains of competence—technical, interpersonal, and critical thinking skills—that are often addressed in literature. Del Bueno developed a performance-based development system (PBDS) that focuses on these three aspects of practice.

The PBDS provides initial assessment data about a nurse's ability to perform and identifies learning needs. Clinical judgment skills are assessed through a series of videotaped patient scenarios in which the nurse must identify the problem and outline what steps should be taken to solve that problem to assess his or her ability to recognize and manage patient problems and give rationale for interventions taken.

Patient kardexes and care plans also provide the opportunity to assess the nurse's ability to prioritize scheduled activities for patients, and event cards are used to assess the nurse's ability to determine the priority for unscheduled events. If a task is a must-do event, the nurse must identify the appropriate action to be taken.

Audiotapes of various nurse–physician or nurse–nurse interactions assess the nurse's ability to recognize ineffective interpersonal strategies and identify interventions that could achieve more desirable outcomes. Some technical skills are demonstrated in a clinical laboratory setting, whereas others are demonstrated on the clinical unit. After the nurse completes the assessment, the assigned clinical instructor completes a profile documenting the assessment, develops an action plan that summarizes the findings, and identifies learning needs. The focus on technical skills, interpersonal skills, and critical-thinking skills is helpful, although the initial evaluation of competence for new hires may be too time-intensive.

Some roles may require competencies in other domains appropriate for those roles. For instance, managers must demonstrate leadership competencies. In our increasingly diverse healthcare environment, it is important for staff members to demonstrate cultural competence when caring for patients of different backgrounds. Cultural competence encompasses not only racial diversity, but also diversity in age, culture, religious beliefs, sexual orientation, and other demographic factors. Cultural competence builds first on an awareness of one's own cultural perspective and then acknowledges the perspectives of another culture on the same issue.

Levels of competency

People function at various levels, and it is important to identify those differences in competencies. Pat Benner, a nurse theorist, differentiated five levels of skill acquisition in her novice-to-expert theory: novice, advanced beginner, competent, proficient, and expert. This book classifies competencies into three levels: beginner, intermediate, and expert.

Levels of performance are often differentiated by the ability to analyze and synthesize information. Beginners have limited exposure to the tasks expected of them and function at a basic level. With time and the development of expertise, they acquire more skills and can identify potential problems and act accordingly—and they reach the intermediate level. Experts have a wealth of knowledge to draw upon and frequently anticipate problems and plan strategies to avoid them.

A competency on performing a respiratory assessment would be a beginning competency for an RN, whereas initiating actions to prevent or minimize complications based on one's assessment data would be an intermediate competency, and appropriately responding to subtle changes in respiratory assessment data would be a more expert competency.

Who performs competency validation?

After identifying expected competencies for each job classification, the next step is to determine who can validate competencies. This role will vary depending on the resources and types of personnel in the facility.

The American Nurses Association's *Nursing: Scope and Standards of Practice* addresses the mandate that nurses must provide care competently and keep up with current nursing practice (ANA 2004). Individuals at all levels of the organization must assume personal responsibility to maintain their competence and ensure that they follow the system established by their organization to validate their competence.

Every organization has a responsibility to ensure that all staff members who provide patient care are educated appropriately and are competent to fulfill their job responsibilities and meet acceptable standards. To meet the requirements of The Joint Commission and other accrediting bodies, organizations must also ensure ongoing competence of employees (Joint Commission Resources 2008). To do this, they must establish a competency system and determine who can validate competence.

Various individuals or groups with documented expertise in an area can validate competence of others. For instance, an agency could determine that either RNs or licensed practical nurses (LPNs) can validate nursing assistants' (NAs') competency in taking vital signs. For lifting and transfer techniques, someone from physical therapy or nurses could validate competency. For some skills, someone in one job category could validate the competence of another person in that same category. For instance, an RN experienced in critical care could validate the competence of a fellow RN in measuring cardiac output.

Organizations must identify clearly who can validate competencies and ensure that they have the appropriate education, experience, or expertise with that skill to perform the competency validation. Anyone who validates competence should be trained to do so (see Chapter 4) and should use an established competency checklist to ensure consistency with the evaluation process (see Chapter 6).

Mandatory training versus competencies

There is often confusion between competencies and mandatory training required by regulatory agencies or institutional policy. Most organizations require that all staff members review a variety of safety topics on a yearly basis, such as fire safety, dealing with emergency situations (e.g., cardiac arrests, disasters, hazardous materials, etc.), and cultural diversity. Institutions have a variety of ways to achieve this task. Some distribute self-learning packets (SLPs) containing the essential information and require everyone to review that material annually. Some SLPs may require that the individual take a posttest, and others may require simply that the individual read the information. Institutions that have computer capabilities may require personnel to complete safety programs online. Some may hold face-to-face sessions, which may or may not include some hands-on practice with the skill, for reviewing the information.

The difference between mandatory training and competency validation is that the latter requires demonstration of the skill, whereas the former does not necessarily do so. To further clarify the difference, the following list outlines some of the common safety topics required by regulatory agencies:

- Cultural competence and ethical conduct
- Privacy and confidentiality issues (e.g., Health Insurance Portability and Accountability Act of 1996 [HIPAA] requirements)
- Fire safety
- Disaster preparedness
- Emergency codes
- Electrical safety
- Infection control and bloodborne pathogens
- Institutional safety plan and patient safety
- Back safety
- Emergency response to various threats (e.g., bombs, patient/family violence)

An example of competency is many organizations' requirement that personnel maintain competence in basic life support (BLS), which requires a staff member to complete appropriate courses as a healthcare provider, heart saver, or advanced cardiac life-support provider.

The focus on competencies is on what the individual can do, not what he or she knows, and competencies must be measured in a simulated or clinical setting. One example of a competency that can be demonstrated without specific patient contact is blood-glucose testing. Any healthcare provider who tests blood sugar results must get an accurate reading because treatment is based on those results. The lab can provide a contrast material to the units so that individuals can run a sample and send their results to the lab. The lab can determine the accuracy of the individual's reading and his or her ability to use the machine correctly by comparing the individual's results with the test material.

Mapping competencies for orientation, annual assessments

You can determine which skills should be evaluated each year in a variety of ways. Selected competencies can be based on the needs of an individual unit, identified quality-improvement needs or problems, changes in patient population, care modalities, or new technologies. Summarized performance appraisal results could be used to indicate the particular competencies staff members need to develop further. Skills that are not used frequently but that present high risk to the patient can also be validated. Most institutions require some safety training annually, as well as BLS courses; these can also be part of the competency process. Many organizations are working toward integrating their performance appraisal and competency management systems. We will discuss this further in Chapter 3.

Some institutions focus on skills that are high-risk, low-volume, or problem-prone (Cooper 2002).

High-risk activities can cause serious (or deadly) damage to a patient or staff member if performed incorrectly. Look at high-risk activities closely. If they are performed every day, they are considered high-volume. High-volume activities do not necessarily need to be reviewed every year, although they should be a part of your orientation program. The assumption is that you perform the activity so often that you know it well.

Low-volume skills are not performed very often within your department, but employees still need to know how to perform them well. These skills should be reviewed at least annually. If an activity is both high-risk and low-volume, you definitely should include it in your annual review.

Problem-prone skills are the subject of unusual occurrence reports or other error reporting forms or quality assurance data. These data should be reviewed regularly, because they are an excellent source of skill or knowledge deficits that become annual competencies. Near misses are also serious enough for a review.

Elizabeth Parsons and Mary Bona Capka suggested a model to determine how frequently skills should be assessed based on risk (Parsons and Capka 1997). Although this may be more detailed than necessary for some organizations, it may be helpful to identify high-risk procedures. The following are the key factors in their model:

- **Incident frequency:** This is determined by a rating scale that includes occurrence, quality improvement, and compliance data. Occurrence scores are ranked on a Likert-type scale (e.g., 5 = daily; 4 = once per week; 3 = once per month; 2 = once in six months; 1 = once per year or less; 0 = never). Incidents are defined as untoward incidents, equipment problems, staff noncompliance, or infection control data reported in the past 12 months. The more incidents, the higher the score.
- **Use/performance frequency:** This identifies the equipment use or competency performance. It uses the same Likert-type scale as the incident frequency scale, but with reversed scoring (e.g., 5 = once per year or less; 1 = daily). If procedures are performed infrequently, important steps may be inadvertently omitted. The more frequently the staff member performs the competency, the lower the score.
- **Patient/operator risk:** This scale scores each item according to the risk to the patient or operator if the competency is performed incorrectly. The highest score (i.e., 5 = operator or patient death) is assigned to competencies for which there is great risk to the patient or staff member, where the lowest score (i.e., 1 = barely any risk) is used if there is no significant risk to the patient or staff member.
- **Skill complexity:** This score captures the skills' complexity and is based on Benner's novice-to-expert model. Skills that the new graduate should be able to perform without supervision would rank lowest (1 or 2), whereas skills that require application of theoretical principles in creative and innovative ways score highest (9 or 10). In this manner, skills necessary to perform an identified competency factor into decisions made about the frequency of assessment.

The formula that Parsons and Capka used captured all these components, with risk being identified as the most crucial factor. Additional weight or value was given to the patient/operator risk score. Their formula appears in the box that follows. Scores range from 0 to 100.

Incident frequency (I) + user frequency (U) + skill complexity (C)
X patient/operator risk (R) = Total score (T), or

$$(I + F + C) R = T$$

For example, a skill such as providing immediate support for a cardiac arrest (e.g., BLS or advanced life support) would have a relatively high risk score. The incident frequency would encompass the number of untoward events during codes in the past year (in this case, 1). User frequency would vary, but for most non-critical-care areas, it would be rated high (a rating of 5) because it is not routinely performed in those areas. Complexity would be rather high (a rating of 8) because a code is a complex patient-care situation, and the risk would be high (a rating of 5) because inappropriate performance of the competency could lead to patient death. A potential score of 70 could be obtained using the formula given earlier: (1 + 5 + 8) 5 = 70.

Your method for mapping competencies to be validated needs to be flexible enough to allow for changes or modifications based on environmental factors. For instance, a new piece of equipment might require the staff to demonstrate competency in using that equipment. The system would need to be flexible enough to include that as an additional competency in a timely manner for the affected staff members.

Methods for validating competencies

It is important to realize that there are numerous ways to validate competencies. One of the most common methods is the skills checklist, which is described in Chapter 6. However, there are many other ways that competence can be validated (Avillion, Brunt, and Ferrell 2007).

Posttests

Posttests are one method for documenting cognitive knowledge and are sometimes used as a method for documenting competence. However, when competency is defined as the overall ability to perform, many tests do not have a performance aspect. One way that tests can be used is to document basic knowledge so that participants don't have to take a course or program when they can show that they have the basic knowledge required in that course. For instance, someone with critical-care experience could take a posttest to document that he or she has sufficient knowledge about a particular skill (e.g., cardiac monitoring) and, as a result, does not have to take that session of the curriculum. However, this would not take the place of validating his or her skills in the clinical area. Some tests may provide a written description, a videotape or audiotape, a live simulation, or printed or projected still pictures, and then present specific questions to which the test taker must respond. Del Bueno's PBDS uses this approach to validate competency.

Observations of daily work

Observations of daily work, such as patient rounds or medical-record reviews, can be a means of validating competency. Specific interactions or skills can be directly observed as someone performs his or her work, and patient outcomes/documentation can be observed as well. This provides an opportunity for multiple observations and addresses one of the problems with checklists, which usually gather data from only one observation of a task. When staff members know they are being observed, they have a tendency to go through all the steps correctly when they might not normally do so.

Case studies

Case studies are another means of validating competency. Individuals can describe how they would provide care for a particular patient or how they would deal with a particular scenario presented to them. These can also be used to address age-specific competencies. After someone describes how he or she would take care of a 37-year-old diabetic patient, the assessor could ask that person what he or she would do differently if the patient was 65 years old. The person's description of the factors he or she would consider and how he or she would alter the patient's care could be used to document the person's ability to care for patients of different ages.

Peer review/360° evaluation

Peer review, or a technique called "360° evaluation," is another method for validating competency. The 360° evaluation incorporates feedback from as many people who interact with a staff member as is feasible. For an RN, these people might include peers, LPNs, NAs, representatives of other disciplines, and the RN's manager. The use of different sources of information and different measures to evaluate competence increases validity.

Exemplars

Exemplars are narrative descriptions of practice. Individuals describe how they handled a particular situation, in essence writing or telling a story about it. Their narrative allows the clinician to describe the step-by-step progression of the incident, as well as the feelings, thoughts, and conclusions from their reflection of the situation. These exemplars can be part of portfolios that can provide concrete examples of competence in a particular area.

Simulated events

Simulated events, such as mock codes, can also be used to validate competency. For example, the instructor can use a mannequin in a bed to describe scenarios and ask the participants to respond appropriately. This provides an opportunity for practice and demonstration of skills in a nonthreatening environment. Another example is the use of volunteers as simulated patients for staff members to perform assessments or demonstrate various noninvasive skills. Also available are various simulators that provide a realistic environment for demonstration of skills, but these can be costly.

Quality-improvement monitors

Quality-improvement monitors, if they reflect individual performance, are another method for validating competency. These are often related to quality-of-care issues such as falls, documentation, healthcare-acquired infections, and so on. With the ongoing emphasis on performance improvement and quality, most organizations have a quality-improvement program and quality monitors in place. For example, an institution may document compliance with the new HIPAA security requirements by having individuals without name tags approach staff members and tell them that they work for IT services. They may ask the employees for their passwords to check the computer system or tell a secretary they are responding to a call about a computer problem and remove a piece of computer equipment from that secretary's manager's office. If the employee does not follow the established policy, feedback and follow-up are provided.

Scheduling and organizing the competencies

Once the competencies to be validated are determined, the organization needs to communicate them to all staff members and provide the tools necessary to validate those skills. This can be done in a variety of ways. Access to the various checklists or methods to validate competencies should be available for all staff members to use during the validation process.

Some organizations may choose to have competency notebooks on each unit that include a tracking sheet of employees and a list of which competencies need validation for each level of personnel. Samples of skills checklists or other methods to validate competencies should also be included in the notebook. If a computer-tracking system is in place, this can be used to map individual- or role-specific competencies. Then the person who performs the validation could enter that information directly into the computer system.

Some organizations may choose to put the responsibility on individuals to make sure they are validated on the required competencies annually. In this case, the individual healthcare worker is responsible for having the appropriate person validate the skill and would be responsible for ensuring that the appropriate documentation was completed. These data can then be used in the individual's performance appraisal.

Some institutions may schedule various competencies to be completed by everyone in a designated time frame (e.g., during the first quarter, or two months before their annual performance appraisal). Others may allow competency validation to be done anytime during the year, as long as it is completed by a designated deadline. Whatever system the organization uses to ensure that competence is validated must be communicated to all staff members, and a mechanism needs to be put in place to ensure that the process is followed.

A final step in the competency validation process is to set up a mechanism for ongoing review and evaluation of the process. Specific questions to be included in an evaluation of a competence assessment system are provided in Chapter 6.

REFERENCES

1. American Nurses Association. (2004). *Nursing: Scope and Standards of Practice.* Washington, DC: ANA.

2. Avillion, Brunt B., and Ferrell M. 2007. *Nursing Professional Development Review and Resource Manual.* Silver Spring, MD: Institute for Credentialing Innovation.

3. Brunt, Barbara A. (2007). *Competencies for Staff Educators: Tools to Evaluate and Enhance Nursing Professional Development.* Marblehead, MA: HCPro, Inc.

4. Cooper, D. (2002). "The 'C' Word: Competency" in Kristen L. O'Shea, *Staff Development Nursing Secrets.* Philadelphia: Hanley & Belfus.

5. Joint Commission Resources. (2008). *Comprehensive Accreditation Manual for Hospitals: The Official Handbook.* Oakbrook Terrace, IL: Joint Commission Resources.

6. Parsons, Elizabeth C., and Mary Bona Capka. (1997.) "Building a successful risk-based competency assessment model." *AORN Journal* 66(6): 1065–1071.

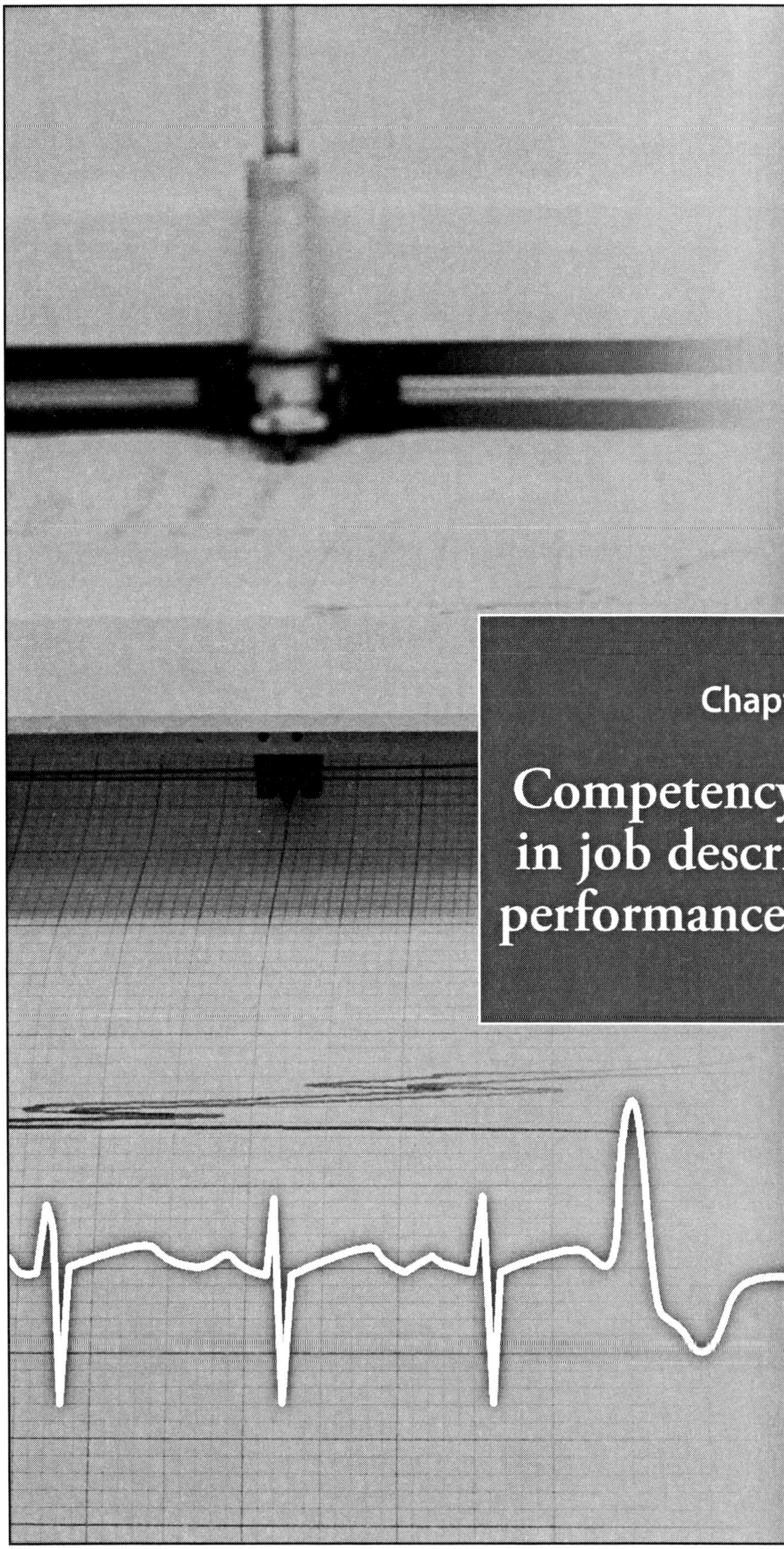

Chapter 3

Competency validation in job descriptions and performance evaluations

Chapter 3

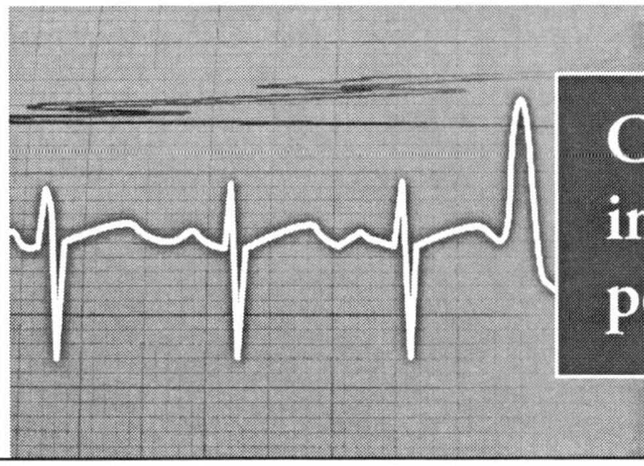

Competency validation in job descriptions and performance evaluations

Learning objectives

After reading this chapter, the participant should be able to:

- Recognize the benefits of incorporating competency assessment into job descriptions and performance evaluation tools
- Discuss the key elements required of performance-based job descriptions

New technology, legislation, and accreditation standards are changing the job responsibilities of those employed at your organization almost every day. In some cases, these forces make it necessary for your organization to create entirely new job positions to keep pace and ensure safe, quality care. As a result, it is more difficult for hospitals to work with HR to keep job descriptions current, create effective and realistic performance evaluations that are in sync with those job descriptions, and include these tools in a process for assessing initial and ongoing competencies.

In this chapter, we will provide further support for the underpinning theme throughout this book: manageability. That is, not only should you make your competency validation and assessment process compliant and effective, but you should also make it manageable. This chapter discusses the elements required to build competency-based job descriptions.

Competency-based (sometimes called performance-based) job descriptions state employee responsibilities in terms of practice standards, or how these responsibilities must be demonstrated, rather than simply listing duties and responsibilities. Competency-based job descriptions, which can double as performance evaluation tools, will also help you meet HR standards set by The Joint Commission.

Although these tools will take a good deal of time to develop, they will help your organization have a more streamlined system for developing performance criteria for your competency validation skill sheets, for assessing age/population-specific competencies, and for tying those assessments into timely performance evaluations. In this chapter, we will discuss:

- The benefits of incorporating competency assessment into your job descriptions and performance evaluation tools
- What The Joint Commission expects from hospitals in this area
- The key elements required of performance-based job descriptions
- Practical tips for complying with The Joint Commission's challenging HR.3.20 standard, which expects timely completion of performance evaluations

The benefits

Your organization can expect several benefits from incorporating competency assessment into its job descriptions and performance evaluations, including the following:

- **Improved efficiency:** As long as you are willing to put the time and effort into building competency-based HR tools, your reward will be a more streamlined, compliant competency assessment process. The performance criteria in your job descriptions can serve as the foundation for your competency validation tools (e.g., skill sheets) and performance evaluations.
- **Improved patient safety:** Defining employees' job responsibilities by widely accepted standards or scopes of practice and holding employees to them will help your organization ensure that patient care is delivered in the safest way possible.
- **Improved employee satisfaction:** Employees need validation from their managers or supervisors about their job performance. They need to know what expectations they have or have not met. Well-developed HR tools composed of measurable performance criteria will make it easier for employees to receive this type of validation.

The Joint Commission's expectations

According to The Joint Commission, one of its competency assessment requirements, HR standard 3.10 (formerly HR5), ranks as the most-cited issue for hospitals accredited by The Joint Commission. HR.3.10 expects that hospitals assess staff competencies in relation to performance expectations outlined in their job descriptions (Joint Commission Resources 2008).

If experience is any measure, it's no wonder organizations struggle with developing effective, time-tested competency assessment tools. In the past, a survey team would visit a facility and make recommendations on how it could improve its competency assessment process or the tools associated with it. The facility would implement modifications based on those recommendations; then, three years later, a different survey team would come in and tell the organization something completely different. As a result, facilities had many different ideas about how to build an effective competency assessment program.

Scenarios such as this one fostered the need for a process, mechanism, or tool to help hospitals develop strong competency assessment programs. A well-developed competency-based job description accomplishes this.

We discussed The Joint Commission's expectations for competency assessment in Chapter 1. As you may recall, the HR.3.10 standard requires that your competency assessment process for staff members, students, and volunteers who work in the same capacity as staff members "providing care, treatment, and services" be based on, above all, populations served and the defined competencies required for each staff member. Therefore, there must be an effort to identify and validate population-specific competencies (which we will discuss in more detail in Chapter 4). Do all healthcare professionals at your facility need to have these competencies validated? No. The Joint Commission specifies that only staff members who provide care, treatment, and services will need to have this done. Your housekeeping staff, for instance, does not need to have population-specific competencies validated.

However, keep in mind that some clinical staff members who aren't licensed will need to have their competencies validated. Pharmacy technicians, for example, are not licensed in many states, yet they fall into the category of clinical staff and deal a lot with medications. Although they're not licensed, pharmacy technicians clearly need to have an understanding of population-specific concerns regarding medication. Dietary aides are another example. They are unlicensed staff members who do not assess or treat patients, but how they deliver food differs based on the type of patient. They may need to have population-specific competencies validated.

The Joint Commission also requires you to define a time frame for how often competency assessments are performed and (in HR.3.20) how often performance evaluations are performed. The Joint Commission says this should be done at least once in the three-year accreditation cycle. Most important, however, is that you meet the objectives and goals associated with the time frame your organization chooses. If you fail to meet your expectations, The Joint Commission will cite you.

This highlights the efficiency and effectiveness of a competency assessment process that incorporates both your job descriptions, which spell out the expectations, accountabilities, and competencies associated with the job, and performance evaluations, which allow managers to provide feedback on a regular basis and track employees' progress toward those expectations, accountabilities, and competencies.

Key elements of a competency-based job description

What makes a job description competency- or performance-based?

The foundation for each employee's job description should be the position's qualifications, duties, and responsibilities. However, well-developed competency- or performance-based job descriptions at your facility must state employee responsibilities (i.e., essential functions and nonessential functions) in terms of expected practice standards—in other words, how the responsibilities must be demonstrated. Created by the department manager and understood by the HR department, these standards must have measurable, objective outcomes associated with them. The problem with many job descriptions is that they are written in a way that leads to subjective interpretations by supervisors.

Include an associated rating scale, which includes definitions that have been agreed upon across departments. This scale must be clear and easy to understand for everyone using it. Also include within job descriptions an area for a supervisor to document in narrative format how the employee met expectations.

All the examples in the following section will be based on the job description of a floating RN, in the medical-surgical unit.

Essential and nonessential functions

Essential functions are those tasks, duties, and responsibilities that compose the context of the job (i.e., the means of accomplishing the job's purpose and objectives). The essential functions should be measurable statements that cover the major components of the job for which the person will be held accountable. Figure 3.1 shows an example of two essential functions and their expected performance criteria.

Functions listed as nonessential aren't unimportant—they just are not critical for the performance of the job position. They should be listed as specifically as possible and also should include performance criteria.

Figure 3.1

Essential functions

1. Assesses and diagnoses patient and family needs to provide quality care to assigned patients.			
Performs admission assessment within eight hours of admission or in accordance with specific unit standards.			
❑ Consistently does not meet standards	❑ Developmental/ Needs improvement	❑ Consistently meets/ sometimes exceeds standards	❑ Consistently exceeds standards
Identifies and documents nursing diagnosis on patients' plan of care within eight hours of admission.			
❑ Consistently does not meet standards	❑ Developmental/ Needs improvement	❑ Consistently meets/ sometimes exceeds standards	❑ Consistently exceeds standards
Identifies and documents patient/family/significant other of admission.			
❑ Consistently does not meet standards	❑ Developmental/ Needs improvement	❑ Consistently meets/ sometimes exceeds standards	❑ Consistently exceeds standards
Overall rating			
❑ Consistently does not meet standards	**❑ Developmental/ Needs improvement**	**❑ Consistently meets/sometimes exceeds standards**	**❑ Consistently exceeds standards**
Performance narrative			

2. Develops, discusses, and communicates a realistic problem list (plan of care) for each patient, in collaboration with each patient/family/significant other in order to address all identified needs.			
Plan of care will include nursing diagnosis statement for each identified problem.			
❑ Consistently does not meet standards	❑ Developmental/ Needs improvement	❑ Consistently meets/ sometimes exceeds standards	❑ Consistently exceeds standards
Develops patient/family/significant other teaching and discharge plan as per unit standard.			
❑ Consistently does not meet standards	❑ Developmental/ Needs improvement	❑ Consistently meets/ sometimes exceeds standards	❑ Consistently exceeds standards
Overall rating			
❑ Consistently does not meet standards	**❑ Developmental/ Needs improvement**	**❑ Consistently meets/sometimes exceeds standards**	**❑ Consistently exceeds standards**
Performance narrative			

Organizational competencies

Job descriptions should also include organizational competencies—those that are expected across all departments of the organization for every employee. This will often require you to incorporate competency-based performance standards in sections devoted to (but not limited to):

- Service
- Teamwork
- Communication
- Respect for others
- Time and priority management
- Mandatory safety requirements
- Leadership competencies

Rating scale and definitions

The rating-scale portion of your job descriptions is extremely important. To develop a rating scale that is agreed upon across the organization, consider:

- How many levels of ratings are required to differentiate performance
- How many standards can be identified, maintained, and discriminated in your performance appraisal process
- The reliability of raters across the organization in judging standards
- Whether the rating scale produces improved performance and communication

An example of a rating scale and definitions appears in Figure 3.2.

Figure 3.2

Rating scale and definitions

Consistently exceeds standards	Performance consistently surpasses all established standards. Activities often contribute to improved innovative work practices. This category is to be used for truly outstanding performance.
Consistently meets/ Sometimes exceeds standards	Performance meets all established standards and sometimes exceeds them. Activities contribute to increased unit/departmental results. Employees consistently complete the work that is required and at times go beyond expectations.
Developmental/Needs improvement	Performance meets most but not all established standards. Activities sometimes contribute to unit/department results. This category is to be used for employees who must demonstrate improvement or more consistent performance and/or for employees still learning their job.
Consistently does not meet standards	Performance is consistently below requirements/expectations. Immediate improvement is necessary.

Performance narratives

Performance narratives offer supervisors an opportunity to document their ongoing feedback and evaluation of staff performance. Your goal should be to establish consistency in rating performance across the organization. There is a lot of disagreement regarding what constitutes a good performance evaluation. However, the general thinking is that if you stick to criteria established in your job descriptions you will make it easier on employees and satisfy Joint Commission surveyors.

To this end, a narrative box can be placed at the end of each essential function in your job description (refer back to Figure 3.1). This differs from most traditional performance evaluations, which have space only at the end of the form to document a narrative. This format would allow a supervisor to apply more specific feedback and recommendations.

Compliance tips for HR.3.20

Timely completion of performance evaluations is critical to the success of your entire organization and your Joint Commission survey. To ensure that success, some organizations have established 30- to 90-day windows from the time the reviews are sent out to the time they are due for managers to get the work done. Here is some more advice from industry experts to reduce your turnaround time and reduce your risk of noncompliance with The Joint Commission's HR.3.20:

1. Keep your performance evaluations realistic. A lot of organizations go to great lengths to design comprehensive performance evaluations that address every potential aspect of competency, but managers can't complete them because they are too complicated, says Bud Pate, REHS, practice director for clinical operations improvement for The Greeley Company, a division of HCPro, Inc., in Marblehead, MA.

2. Post reminders. The key to success is discipline, according to Glenn D. Krasker, MHSA, president of Critical Management Solutions, a consulting firm that specializes in medical error risk reduction, in Wilmington, DE. It's best if evaluations are due on employee anniversary dates, rather than all of the organization's evaluations being due on the same date, so the workload is spread out over 12 months.

3. Institute self-evaluations. Help to reduce the burden on supervisors by getting employees to complete a self-assessment of their job performance prior to the performance evaluation, which the manager will amend before it is sent to HR, says Katherine Chamberlain, CPHQ, a consultant in Gloucester, MA.

4. Hold supervisors accountable. Tie in supervisors' evaluations and pay increases to the timelines of their completion of staff evaluations, suggests Krasker.

5. Condense your evaluations. Make sure your evaluations are not overly burdensome. Try to keep the document to one or two pages, says Pate.

6. Automate the process. Online performance evaluation tools help to streamline the process because the forms are easily accessible to everyone and can be filled out quickly and legibly, says Deb Ankowicz, RN, BSN, CPHQ, director of risk management for the University of Wisconsin Hospitals & Clinics, in Madison.

7. Have a blitz day. If managers are running behind schedule, reserve a conference room where they can work without interruptions to get their evaluations done, says Krasker.

Source: Adapted from ***Briefings on The Joint Commission newsletter****, published by HCPro, Inc.*

The key to successfully incorporating your competency assessment process into the ongoing maintenance of job descriptions and the completion of performance evaluations is to develop manageable tools. At the very least, these tools need to identify measurable performance criteria and promote consistent, agreed-upon methods for evaluating the staff (based in part on the populations with which they work) and getting it all done in a timely manner.

REFERENCES

1. Joint Commission Resources. (2008). *Comprehensive Accreditation Manual for Hospitals: The Official Handbook*. Oakbrook Terrace, IL: Joint Commission Resources.

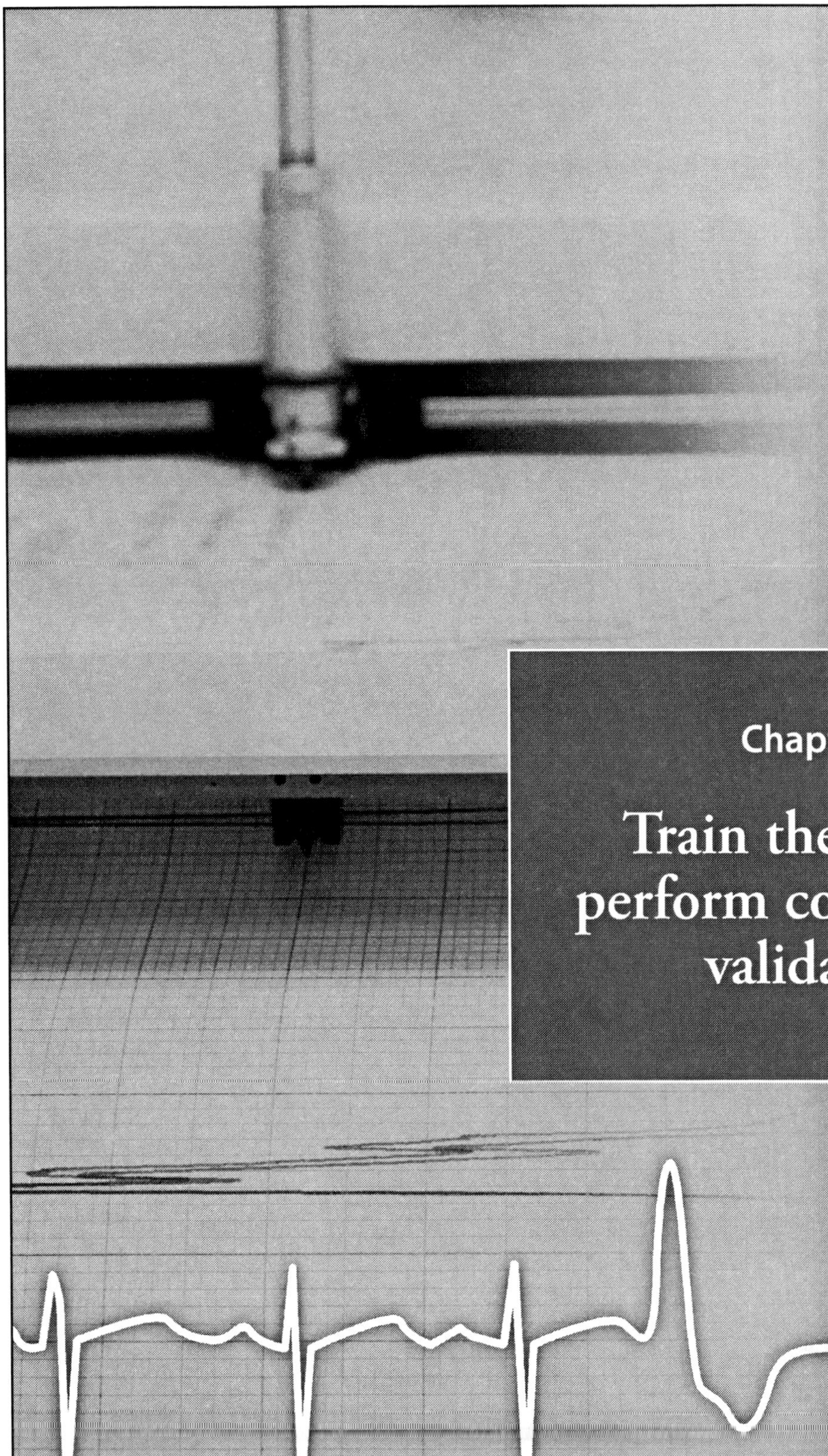

Chapter 4

Train the staff to perform competency validation

Chapter 4

Train the staff to perform competency validation

Learning objectives

After reading this chapter, the participant should be able to:

- Develop a training program to train staff to perform competency assessment
- Maintain consistency in a competency validation system
- Identify steps for effective program documentation
- Recognize the essential qualities needed by competency assessors

Who performs competency validation within your organization? How are they trained to perform this important responsibility? Ideally, those who assess the competency of others are selected based on their clinical skills and ability to help colleagues enhance job performance. This means they also possess tact and good teaching skills and receive appropriate training prior to evaluating colleagues' job performance. The opposite of this ideal situation is to have all staff members assess the competency of others with little or no training, regardless of their teaching skills.

The truth is, most organizations fall somewhere between these two extremes. The purpose of this chapter is to help you design a practical training program for those staff members responsible for assessing the competency of others.

Developing a competency assessment training program

Who should be trained to perform competency assessment? First, understand that not all staff members should be trained to assess their colleagues' competency. Competency assessment is an acquired skill that not all healthcare professionals possess.

What qualifications should a competency assessor possess?

- Excellent performance of the competencies being evaluated
- Tact and the desire to help colleagues improve their job performance
- The desire to acquire/enhance adult education skills
- Demonstration of excellent interpersonal communication skills

Now that you know who should be trained, what should you include in the training program? The following components should be part of your competency assessment training and education program.

Purpose

Learners need to understand the purpose and importance of a competency assessment program. You need to be able to demonstrate how job performance is enhanced and patient care improved by adhering to competency criteria. Use quality improvement and risk management data to prove your point. Learners must also understand that The Joint Commission and other accrediting agencies expect staff members to demonstrate their competence, that such competence is evaluated on an ongoing basis, and that each staff member's competence is documented.

Principles of adult learning

Any education program that involves training adults to teach/coach other adults must include an overview of the principles of adult learning (Avillion, Brunt, and Ferrell 2007).

- **Adults must have a valid reason for learning.** Adults want proof that there is a need for learning (i.e., they want to know why it is important for them to participate in an educational activity). For example, suppose the ability to draw arterial blood gases is a competency for all RNs on the medical ICU. Some of them complain that they perform this task frequently and they don't need someone observing them to validate their competency. If you are able to cite quality improvement data indicating a negative trend (e.g., infections, bruising, etc.) due to questionable techniques, you can show them why there is a need for continual competency assessment. National data can also be cited to illustrate the need for keeping "on top" of a particular skill.

- **Adults are self-directed learners.** Adults direct their own learning. They want to feel that they have some control over what they learn and the manner in which they learn it. Adults also need to feel that their opinions matter and their learning needs are respected.

- **Adults bring a variety of life experiences to any learning situation.** Such life experiences can facilitate any learning activity. Even experiences not directly related to healthcare can enhance education.

- **Adults concentrate on acquiring knowledge and skills that help them improve their professional and/or personal lives.** Adults measure the importance of education by focusing on how new knowledge and skills will help them improve their professional performance or enhance their private lives.

- **Adults respond to both extrinsic and intrinsic motivators.** Adults must know how learning activities meet their extrinsic and intrinsic needs. Extrinsic motivators include things such as job promotions and raises in salaries. Examples of intrinsic motivators include enhanced self-esteem and an increase in job satisfaction.

Learning styles

When you assess competency, you are often in the position of teacher. Even though a staff member demonstrates competency, you may have suggestions to help improve some aspect of his or her skill. Include an overview of learning styles when you design your competency assessment training program (Avillion 2004):

- **Auditory learners:** Auditory learners assimilate knowledge by hearing. They prefer lectures, discussions, and audiotapes. They respond most favorably to verbal instructions.

- **Visual learners:** Visual learning is the most predominant adult learning style. Visual learners sit in the front of a classroom, take detailed notes, and respond to verbal discussions that contain large amounts of imagery.

- **Kinesthetic learners:** Kinesthetic learners learn best by "doing." They need direct hands-on involvement and physical activity as part of the learning experience.

Maintaining objectivity

It is important that those who assess competency maintain their objectivity. The training program should contain information about performing objective evaluations and not letting personal feelings—positive or negative—influence the outcome of the assessment.

Offering constructive criticism

This is one of the most challenging responsibilities of anyone who evaluates the job performance of others. The purpose of constructive criticism is to provide feedback on both strengths and weaknesses. Constructive criticism should motivate, reinforce learning, and identify the nature and extent of problems. One of the most important parts of constructive criticism is the development of a specific plan to help staff members improve their performance. Use the following four steps when giving feedback:

1. **Identify the unacceptable actions.** What is the staff member doing or failing to do that is not acceptable? Remember to focus on the employee's behavior, *not* on his or her personality. Give specific examples, such as "You did not follow sterile techniques when you touched the IV tubing with your sterile-gloved hand," not "It seems as though you do not care whether you endanger the patient by ignoring proper sterile techniques."

2. **Explain the outcome.** What about the behavior is unacceptable? How does it negatively impact productivity, patient outcomes, and so on? Be specific. Use descriptive terms instead of evaluative terms.

3. **Establish the expectation.** What must the employee do to correct unacceptable behavior? Again, be specific, and use objective, descriptive terms. You are describing actions to improve behavior, not providing evaluative comments about a person's personality.

4. **Identify the consequences.** What will happen if the employee corrects his or her behavior? What will happen if he or she does not?

How to assess competency consistently

One of the biggest challenges of any competency assessment program is the need for consistency among those conducting the assessments. How do you make sure that one person is not too stringent and another too lenient? Are friends assessing friends' competency? Does this make a difference in the outcome? Are people who dislike each other assessing each other's competency? Your training program must provide staff members with the tools and support needed to conduct competency assessments properly. This includes maintaining up-to-date policies and procedures, appropriate documentation checklists, and adequate education and training (a detailed description of these components appears later in this chapter).

Consistency in documentation is as important as consistency in approach. Everyone should use the same tool template. A procedure that describes how to document competency is needed.

Identifying your competency assessors

Can you identify competency assessors by title? Let's look at some common job titles that may carry with them the responsibility for competency assessment.

- **Preceptors:** The ability to perform competency assessment is an integral part of the preceptor role. The preceptor is necessary to the successful orientation of new employees. The essential qualities needed by competency assessors are also preceptor attributes. These qualities include the following:
  - Possesses excellent clinical skills or, in nonclinical roles, excellence in job-specific skills
  - Demonstrates respect for colleagues
  - Acts as an excellent role model
  - Demonstrates outstanding interpersonal communication skills

  The assumption that preceptors adequately assess competency is based on the belief that your preceptor training program includes the essential components described earlier in this chapter. To increase the efficiency of training delivery, consider inviting staff members who need to be trained as competency assessors (but who are not preceptors) to the preceptor classes that offer training in competency assessment.

- **Nurse managers:** Nurse managers are generally not the best people to assess clinical competency. In today's healthcare environment, nurse managers spend the majority of their time performing administrative duties such as staffing, budgeting, developing leadership, and handling performance issues. Their expertise in these areas, however, makes them able to validate such competencies in fellow nurse managers. Nurse managers rely on their staff members to possess clinical expertise, just as staff members rely on nurse managers for administrative expertise. Remember that to assess clinical competency properly, the evaluator must be able to demonstrate excellence in clinical skills. Nurse managers assess the managerial competency of their peers.

- **Staff development specialists:** Staff development specialists are the education experts within a healthcare organization. Their specific roles and areas of expertise determine whether they are involved in clinical competency assessment. For example, a staff development specialist based on the coronary-care unit who provides direct patient care as well as staff education is qualified to assess clinical competency. However, the staff development specialist who primarily offers management and leadership training and does not provide direct patient care is generally not qualified to assess clinical competency.

  Don't forget that staff development specialists must demonstrate competency in the adult education arena as well. Such competencies as program planning, teaching, and evaluating the effectiveness of education are essential to those who specialize in staff development.

  Staff development specialists work with management and the staff to design the organization's entire competency assessment program in addition to the program's training component. They provide the educational expertise that makes for a sound foundation for any competency program. But like anyone else who is responsible for assessing competency, staff development specialists must be competent in the skills that they evaluate.

- **Staff nurses:** Staff nurses who demonstrate the necessary skills may also be part of a competency assessment program. It is important that they receive the necessary training. Depending on the arrangement of your clinical ladder or other similar programs, you may choose to have competency assessment as part of the requirements for promotion.

- **Nursing assistants (NAs):** Can you think of exceptionally competent NAs in your organization? Training such NAs to assess the competency of their peers is a definite possibility. As you develop a promotional ladder for NAs, consider training those who are exceptional to participate in competency assessment.

- **Nonclinical staff:** Most healthcare organizations have competency assessment programs in place for nonclinical areas as well as for clinical areas. As your competency program develops and expands, don't forget to be on the lookout for nonclinical staff members who have what it takes to assess the competency of others.

You already know that you need to document competency achievement. Don't forget to document that your trainees have achieved competency in their ability to evaluate the performance of others. Figure 4.1 shows an example of a form that you can use for such documentation.

Figure 4.1

Successful completion of competency assessment training form

Date: ____________________
Objectives: ____
____
____

Competency demonstration:

1. Explains purpose and importance of a competency assessment program
2. Incorporates the principles of adult learning as part of assessing competency
3. Recognizes various learning styles and meets the needs of learners representing these styles
4. Maintains objectivity when assessing competency
5. Offers feedback in a constructive manner
6. Is consistent in competency assessment approach
7. Documents results of competency assessment accurately and consistently

Trainer comments:
____
____
____

Learner comments:
____
____
____

Competency assessment training was successfully completed:

______________________________ ______________________________
Trainer's signature and date Learner's signature and date

Competency assessment training was not successfully completed:

____
Trainer's signature and date

The following steps will be taken by the learner to successfully complete training:

Action To be completed by the following date:
____
____
____

____
Learner's signature and date

Peer review

The word *peer* is defined as a person or thing having the same rank, value, and/or ability—in other words, an equal. If an important part of your competency program is the concept of "peer review," be careful that you are truly asking peers to evaluate peers. For example, suppose City Hospital's competency policy/procedure states that competency is assessed via a peer-review competency assessment program. City Hospital also has a career ladder for nurses that includes the following titles: staff nurse I, staff nurse II, and staff nurse III.

During a recent competency evaluation session, a staff nurse III (Carolyn) observes a staff nurse II (Amanda) performing the insertion of an intravenous needle. Carolyn documents that Amanda is not competent and needs remedial work. Amanda files a grievance with the hospital disciplinary board stating that Carolyn evaluated her unfairly. In part, the grievance reads, "As a staff nurse III, Carolyn held Amanda to a higher standard, instead of evaluating her according to her experience at the staff nurse II level. Because City Hospital maintains that competency assessment is a form of peer review, Amanda was unfairly evaluated." The disciplinary board supports Amanda, and Carolyn's competency assessment documentation is removed from Amanda's file.

Sound far-fetched? Unfortunately, this kind of problem is not uncommon. Let's look at some pitfalls that might have contributed to City Hospital's (and Carolyn's) dilemma. Consider the following questions/comments:

- Did the policy/procedure clearly define the concept of peer review? Could this problem have been avoided by stating that competency is assessed by several types of staff members (i.e., peers and those functioning at a higher level according to the organization's career ladder)? If the policy is written in this manner, Carolyn could assess the competency of peers, subordinates, and those at a lower level than she on the clinical ladder as long as she is competent in the skill being assessed.

- Did Carolyn receive appropriate training in how to assess competency? Are the results of this training documented?

- Was it clear what had to be accomplished for competency to be achieved? Were the steps in writing and were they part of the competency assessment documentation tool? Did both nurses clearly understand what had to be demonstrated?

- Was objectivity maintained? Do interpersonal conflicts exist between Carolyn and Amanda?

Peer review is an excellent means of support and a worthwhile component of competency assessment. But be very careful that you define what you mean by a peer review. As in the case of City Hospital, if you fail to allow a more experienced nurse to evaluate a less experienced nurse or a subordinate, you may encounter serious problems. You may want to incorporate the definitions of various levels of expertise within your policies and procedures. Use the criteria established by your clinical ladder programs to delineate what levels of the staff are able to evaluate other levels of the staff. It may sound like a lot of extra work or that you're being overcautious, but this type of anticipatory planning prevents or reduces the number of grievances or union actions you encounter.

Keeping your validation system consistent

Nothing is as demoralizing as inconsistency in evaluation, and few things are as challenging as ensuring consistency of approach among many different people. Here are some tips for helping to maintain inter-rater reliability among your competency assessors:

- Select your competency assessor based on the characteristics described earlier in this chapter. You may be tempted to have all members of the nursing staff assess the competency of others. In this day and age of nursing shortages and the need for complex nursing interventions, having everyone assess competency may seem like a quick fix to the problem of documenting competency assessment, but don't succumb to this temptation. In the long run, it will lead to disgruntled employees, failure to adequately assess competency, and a plethora of union and disciplinary grievances. Establish your criteria for selection, put it in writing in policies and procedures, and stick to it.

- The ability to assess the competency of fellow employees is in itself a competency. Successful completion of the training program on competency assessment must be documented. Failure to successfully complete the program demands that the trainee perform remedial work. He or she must not assess the competency of others until training is successfully completed.

- Avoid compromising objectivity whenever possible. If competency is assessed individually in an on-the-job environment, avoid pairing staff members who have known interpersonal conflicts. Likewise, avoid pairing staff members who are close friends. Either situation runs the risk of accusations of favoritism or prejudice. Consider having staff members from other units evaluate each other. Doing so may enhance objectivity.

- Ensure that the steps that must be performed, along with descriptions regarding how they are to be performed, are clearly documented on the competency assessment form. Never assume that "everyone knows how to do this"! Failure to achieve competency can have dramatic consequences, including termination of employment. The only way to ensure consistency fairly is to provide a written guide delineating what constitutes successful competency demonstration.

- Develop a written checklist so that competency is evaluated on a step-by-step basis. The competency assessor must sign and date the checklist. The learner must also sign and date the checklist. Any remedial action plans must be documented along with targeted dates for achievement.

- The person assessing competency must document his or her evaluation findings. This task cannot be delegated to someone else. For example, suppose a busy manager asks one of her senior staff nurses to document a competency assessment for her. This is completely unacceptable. Competency assessment is just like any other type of nursing documentation: You do it, you document it.

- Have a plan in place to deal with persons who object to their competency rating. Include this plan in your policies and procedures. If a staff member is unfairly evaluated, he or she needs to know that there is a professional way to seek a reassessment. The steps that must be taken, including any necessary objective evidence, should be described in these policies and procedures.

- Policies and procedures must also describe the circumstances under which a grievance or other protest mechanism will be heard.

Incorporating population-specific competencies

The Joint Commission changed its focus from age-specific to population-specific care. However, it does not define this term, but leaves it up to the individual institution to do so.

According to Webster's (Agnes 2006), the term *population-specific competency* might be defined as follows:

Population – a. all the people in a country, region, etc. b. a specified part of the people in a given area. c. the total set of persons.

Specific – a. limiting or limited; precise. b. a characteristic of something. c. a special or particular kind.

Competency – a. condition or quality of being competent. b. sufficient for one's needs.

The various physiological and psychological needs of each patient population group is part of any well-designed competency program. The ability to implement population-appropriate interventions is critical to the quality and suitability of patient care.

Most organizations serve a variety of populations and age ranges that can and often do require complex coordination and integration of care. Patient care is managed by staff members who are competent to address the needs of the patient population they serve; whether through case management which targets high-risk populations because of their various combinations of health, social, and functional problems, or through disease management which targets populations that generally have one major diagnosis and a relatively standard set of needs.

Many patient care units are designed based on specialty or specific patient populations. Patients are admitted to units where staff members are familiar with and competent to care for a select patient population as a result of their general, divisional, and unit/population-specific orientations and ongoing education/training and competency assessment. For example, patients requiring total hip replacement will most likely be admitted to an orthopedic unit, those with psychiatric disorders to a behavioral health unit, multiple-trauma patients to an ICU, high-risk pregnancy patients to the perinatal unit, and the list goes on. However, sometimes the complexity of a patient's care requires the skill and competence of a staff trained in several different specialties, necessitating collaboration among various interdisciplinary team members. Figure 4.2 includes examples of population-specific care.

Figure 4.2

Case Studies

A 20-year-old 7-month pregnant woman was admitted to the Perinatal Unit with preeclampsia. Staff members working in this area have been specifically educated and skilled to care for pregnant women with this condition. Unfortunately, the patient did not respond to treatment, convulsed and underwent an emergency cesarean section for the delivery of a healthy baby girl. Clinical and laboratory studies revealed the onset of HELLP syndrome. Within a short period of time the patient became very unstable, requiring a transfer to the ICU. The ICU is staffed by those who have specialized education and skills to meet the needs of this now critically ill adult who required mechanical ventilation and placement of various monitoring devices that can only be used in critical care. For the next 10 days the ICU staff provided the bulk of this patient's care with frequent consultation and input into the plan of care provided by the Mother-Baby staff. Meanwhile the Special Care Nursery staff cared for the infant girl. On day 8, the patient showed much improvement and was transferred to the Mother-Baby unit and finally discharged to home.

A 45-year-old woman with a history of psychiatric problems is admitted for management of a schizophrenic episode. While obtaining her health history, it is discovered that this patient underwent a gastric bypass procedure 6 months ago. She is unable to give a description of the surgical procedure or her current diet to the nurse admitting her. The nurse makes the admitting psychiatrist aware of the recent weight loss surgery procedure. The psychiatrist orders a consult from a Bariatric Surgeon and from the Bariatric Dietitian. The unit secretary calls the Bariatric Care Center to initiate the consult to the surgeon and to the dietitian. The Bariatric Surgeon completes the consult, and talks with the psychiatrist about the impact of the gastric bypass surgery on absorption of medications in the small intestine. The dietitian also sees the patient, and she contacts the dietary staff to make them aware that this patient requires a specific gastric bypass diet. She provides education to the staff regarding the surgery and the reason that this diet is needed, and she makes sure that the orders are entered correctly. She also makes certain that the patient's nurse understands how to verify that the tray is correct when it arrives on the floor. A copy of the consult is provided by the surgeon to the Bariatric Case Manager for the patient's outpatient chart, and the dietitian writes a note in the inpatient chart and the outpatient chart each time she sees the patient. The surgeon requests that the patient be seen in the Bariatric Care Center for follow-up within two weeks of discharge from the hospital.

A 19-year-old male arrives at Same Day Surgery according to standard protocol to undergo gastric bypass surgery. He is extremely obese, with a weight of almost 500 pounds, and arrangements were made in advance for a Hillrom Total Care bed. Upon arrival in the OR, the surgical coordinator observes that the Total Care bed is not available. Knowing that all bariatric patients who exceed 350 pounds must be placed on the Total Care bed, she contacts Distribution to have the bed delivered right away. The

Figure 4.2

Case Studies (cont.)

staff in Distribution, who are also aware of the policy for use of the Total Care bed with bariatric surgery patients, make sure that the bed is taken to the OR within 30 minutes so that it is ready for the patient upon completion of surgery. The patient is moved to the bed while still in the OR, and is ultimately transferred to the inpatient unit on the correct bed. The following morning, again according to protocol, an Upper GI study is ordered for 7:30 am. Upon arrival on the floor, the transporter realizes that the wheelchair he brought is the standard size, and will not accommodate this patient. He thoughtfully does not make note of this in front of the patient, but knowing that there must not be a delay in getting this patient to radiology, goes to the desk and calls down to his department to have a bariatric wheelchair brought up immediately. Another member of the Transportation Department arrives in 15 minutes with a wheelchair, which is appropriate for transportation of a patient of this size, and the patient is safely delivered to Radiology on time for his procedure.

Source: Summa Health System Hospital, Akron, OH. Reprinted with permission.

The demonstration and corresponding documentation of population-specific staff competencies are important for a number of reasons. First, such competency validates the knowledge and skills of staff members. Appropriate knowledge and skills contribute to the quality of patient care and family services. And finally, The Joint Commission requires that population-specific competency be assessed on an ongoing basis and that the findings of these assessments are documented and maintained as part of the employee's file.

Population-specific competency requires proof of education and training, as well as the demonstration of skill achievement. During orientation, all employees must receive education and training concerning the specific patient age groups for which they will provide care. Remember that this includes employees who, although not new to your organization, are new to a department or unit. For example, suppose that Martha has worked on an adult oncology unit for five years. She is transferring to a pediatric oncology unit this month. During Martha's orientation to pediatric oncology, the organization must provide her with education and training specific to pediatric oncology patients. This education and training must be documented and maintained in Martha's employee file.

Does population-specific competency mean that all caregivers must demonstrate competency of all types of patients? No, this is not the case. Identify the age range of patients that staff members encounter most frequently in their work.

For example, a nurse who works on an adult oncology unit cares for patients in the young adult through geriatric age ranges. She or he must demonstrate competency in providing nursing care to patients who are young adults, middle-aged adults, and geriatric adults. Likewise, a nurse who works in a neonatal ICU would need to demonstrate competency in providing care for neonates, not geriatric patients.

What are some efficient, cost-effective ways to achieve and demonstrate population-specific competencies? Let's start with education and training.

Simply attending an education program does not guarantee transfer of learning to the work setting. However, because healthcare science and research seems to bring new and exciting discoveries to the healthcare arena every day, part of the requirement of competency maintenance may involve participating in a specified number of age-specific education hours. These hours do not need to be offered exclusively in a classroom setting. Options such as self-learning packets, videos, and computer-based learning are cost-effective, efficient ways to deliver education and training. Successful achievement of educational posttests measures learning or the acquisition of knowledge.

But as we discussed earlier in this chapter, knowledge acquisition does not equate to the ability to successfully transfer knowledge. How can we assess population-specific competencies? Ongoing competency may be evaluated in several ways, including direct observation, medical record review, and patient outcomes. Let's review the competency of Melanie, a nurse who works on an adult medical-surgical unit. What methodologies can we use to be sure that she is competent in providing care to geriatric patients?

- **Medical record review:** Are appropriate skin care nursing interventions documented? Is there documented evidence that safety measures are in place considering the patient's diagnosis? Has skin turgor been assessed? Identify specific interventions for the assessor to find within the medical record, including nursing care plans, nurses' notes, and so on. You need to be specific to facilitate consistency of evaluation.

- **Direct observations:** Does Melanie provide care in a manner that incorporates age-specific concerns for the geriatric patient? In addition to observing Melanie as she actually provides care, you can assess patient outcomes and the environment. For instance, when assessing safety issues, determine whether the call bell is within reach, whether nonskid slippers are readily available, and so on. Again, be specific about what assessors need to evaluate. Select some universal geriatric issues and determine whether these issues are part of the patient's plan of care.

- **Equipment use:** Is equipment use adapted to the needs of the geriatric patient? For instance, if a geriatric patient is receiving intravenous hydration, are measures taken to avoid fluid overload, a potential danger for an elderly patient?

These are only a few of the ways to assess age related competency. Remember that all reviewers must carry out such assessments in a consistent manner. This means that written guidelines must be established.

Documentation and recordkeeping

It is essential that your competency assessment program include appropriate documentation and maintenance of such documentation. Various sample checklists and templates are presented throughout this chapter. As a summary of important issues, let's review documentation components that are absolutely essential:

- **Assessment documentation must be dated.** Although you may think that this component is self-evident, it is astonishing how many times it is missed. The top of any form generally contains a space for the date, but all signatures should be dated as well. This decreases the chance of any discrepancies concerning assessment dates.

- **Identify the specific competency being assessed.** This includes the specific age ranges assessed as part of age-specific competencies.

- **Identify the objectives that must be achieved to demonstrate competency.** These objectives should be written in measurable terms and contain action verbs such as *performs, identifies, demonstrates*, and so forth. Nonmeasurable terms such as *understand, be aware of*, and so forth are to be avoided.

- **Document specific steps in competency achievement.** Consistency cannot be ensured unless the specific, step-by-step actions that must be performed to achieve competency are in writing. All assessors must have the same expectations of the people they are evaluating.

- **Document the methods used to assess competency.** Possible methods include observation of direct patient care, medical record review, and evaluation of the patient's environment. Again, don't forget to identify what the assessor must look for in the selected method(s).

- **Document remedial action.** If competency is not achieved, document the remedial actions that will be taken to help the learner achieve competency. The actions should be specific and should include target achievement dates.

Conclusion

Competency assessment is an integral part of your patient-care delivery system. Those who assess the competency of others must receive appropriate education and training so that they are effective, efficient, and consistent in their approach.

Careful, objective documentation of such education and training is as important as documentation of competency assessment itself. In fact, achievement as a competency assessor is a competency too. Select with care those individuals who assess competency. Not every staff member is suited to assess and facilitate learning in others. Clinical excellence does not equate to the ability to facilitate the job performance of colleagues.

The templates and forms presented in this chapter are intended to be starting points for the customization of your own tools. Adapt them to meet the needs of your staff members.

Finally, remember that competency assessment is a learning tool as well as a means of validation. Use these opportunities to facilitate the continuing education and professional development of staff members, with the ultimate goal being improved patient outcomes.

REFERENCES

1. Agnes, Michael. (Ed). (2006). *Webster's New World College Dictionary*. Cleveland: Wiley Publishing.

2. Avillion, Adrianne E. (2004). *A Practical Guide to Staff Development: Tools and Techniques for Effective Education*. Marblehead, MA: HCPro, Inc.

3. Avillion, Adrianne E., Barbara Brunt, and Mary Jane Ferrell. (2007). *Nursing Professional Development Review and Resource Manual*. Silver Spring, MD: Institute for Credentialing Innovation.

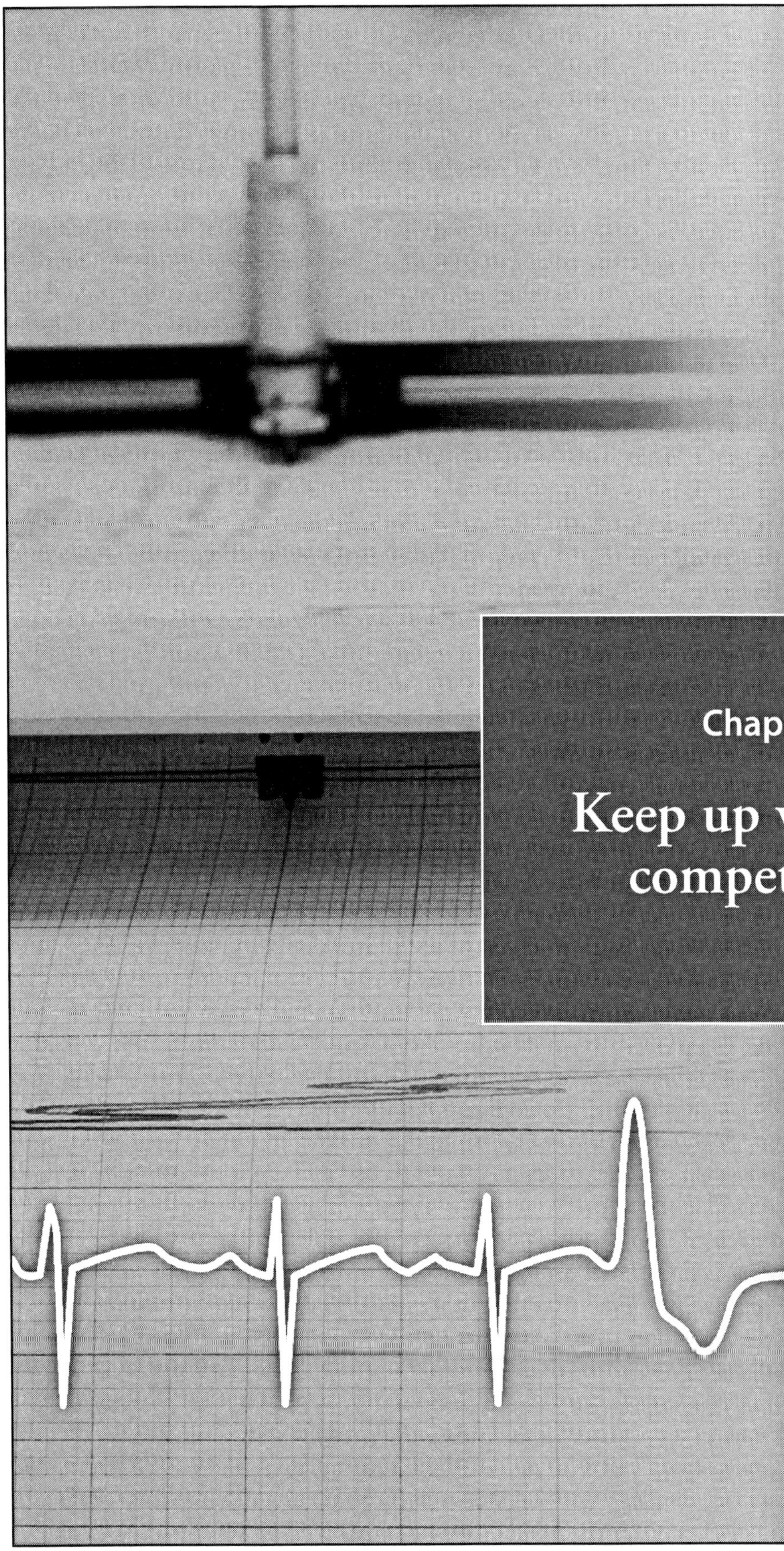

Chapter 5

Keep up with new competencies

Chapter 5

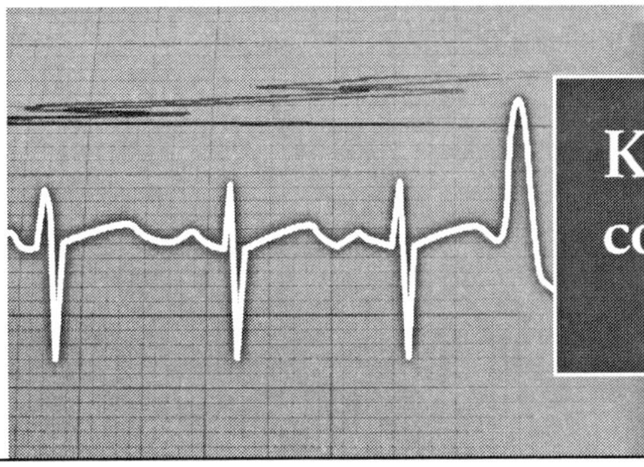

Keep up with new competencies

Learning objectives

After reading this chapter, the participant should be able to:

- List potential categories for new competencies
- Identify best practices for implementing new competencies
- Discuss dimensions of competencies

Hundreds of new concerns arise in healthcare daily. How do you determine which ones become competencies?

Let's start by describing what a competency is not. Competencies are not required for every new piece of equipment, every new or revised policy and procedure, every interpersonal communication problem, or every skill that accompanies a specific job description. However, a competency is a skill that significantly affects or has the potential to significantly affect the patient. Such issues may fall under the categories of psychomotor skills or interpersonal skills.

Doesn't everything in healthcare have the potential to significantly affect a patient? Technically, yes. But if you define the word *significant* that broadly, you will have so many competencies that you'll drown in paperwork, and it will become impossible to assess that many items efficiently.

Potential categories for new competencies

Let's look at some general categories that have the potential for competency development.

New equipment

Not every piece of new equipment triggers the need for a competency. In most cases, a simple inservice suffices. For example, suppose your organization orders new patient beds. The beds have some additional features that the old beds lacked, and an inservice is conducted to orient staff members to work safely with these new beds. Now suppose that new equipment including Circoelectric beds, Bradford frames, and Stryker frames arrives for your organization's newly opened rehabilitation unit. These devices require special skills to ensure patient safety and will be used often, although not daily. These types of new equipment are more suitable for ongoing competency development. They have significant patient impact, require a high level of skill and safety awareness, and are in frequent use.

When new equipment arrives, ask yourself these questions:

- Does the equipment require high levels of skill to operate?
- Who will operate the new equipment? Must the staff have special qualifications (e.g., RN designation) to use this equipment?
- What potential patient safety risks are associated with the new equipment?
- How often will the new equipment be in use?

If you find that equipment requires qualified staff members to have high levels of skill, is associated with significant patient safety issues, and is used often enough that the staff is able to maintain competency, the equipment may require the development of a competency.

Interpersonal communications

Interpersonal communications are the foundation of healthcare interventions. From the first contact at a reception desk or admission's office through and including communication with physicians, nurses, and therapists, interpersonal interaction influences the patient's healthcare experience.

How would you rate interpersonal communication skills among your colleagues? Does risk management/quality improvement data indicate any negative trends in this arena? Do staff members encounter hostility from patients/families? This is not uncommon, especially in areas such as the emergency department, head trauma unit, and inpatient mental health unit. But how do you assess this type of competency? It is not a step-by-step psychomotor skill. However, there are options.

Direct observation is one such option. Keep in mind, however, that written guidelines are necessary for the person assessing competency. Additional observations may be set up in a "competency skills lab" where staff members must respond to various types of behavior in role-play situations. These are not conducted in the actual work setting, but they may be a useful addendum to direct observation.

Be creative when assessing nontechnical skills such as these. Another validation option is to conduct mock drills involving staff members playing the role of agitated/violent patients or family members. These have the advantage of surprise and may be more valuable than a controlled role-play situation.

New patient populations

The appearance of new diseases and syndromes requires the implementation of new diagnostic and treatment interventions. The AIDS epidemic changed almost every aspect of healthcare and triggered the need for universal precautions and more secure protective equipment. The development of new drugs to combat this syndrome requires that healthcare professionals add to the ever-growing body of knowledge concerning medications, their actions, and potential side effects. Similarly, until recently, few healthcare professionals had ever heard of severe acute respiratory syndrome (also known as SARS). Now it is a household term.

The point is that new patient populations require new knowledge and the application of that knowledge in the healthcare setting. As you evaluate the need for new skills to apply this knowledge, you are also evaluating the need for additional competency development. However, stick to the recommendations made earlier in this chapter. Consider the level of knowledge and skill needed, how often the knowledge will be applied, and the effect of these newly acquired skills on patient outcomes.

New treatment measures

Thanks to intense research and scientific inquiry, we are able to treat and even cure illnesses and catastrophic injuries that were untreatable just a few short years ago. With these healthcare advances come new bodies of knowledge and the need to use that knowledge safely and efficiently. As new treatment measures become necessary to your organization's ability to provide patient services, so does the need for additional competency development.

Remember that you don't need to keep the same competencies forever. Perhaps new treatments and equipment and the demise or reduction of certain illnesses (e.g., polio) trigger the need for you to delete certain competencies from your program. As you evaluate the need for new competencies, don't forget to evaluate the need to streamline those already in existence.

New medications

The U.S. Food and Drug Administration approves significant numbers of new medications annually. Most of them do not require competency development; however, some drugs require special knowledge, and administration techniques for these drugs necessitate competency development. Use your guidelines of skill level, patient impact, and frequency of use to determine the need for new competencies.

Research endeavors

If your organization is a research site, your staff members may be exposed to new (and sometimes dangerous) ways of treating illnesses and injuries more often than the average healthcare worker. Examine your research policies and procedures. Which staff members frequently initiate experimental treatments, including medication administration? How do you measure their competency to initiate these treatments? As you evaluate your competency assessment program, don't forget to pay close attention to the research conducted at your organization: The resultant treatment initiatives could mandate the development of new competencies.

Guidelines for new competency development

Develop a policy that guides your competency assessment program (Avillion 2004). Part of that policy describes your guidelines for new competency development (and for the deletion of competencies that are no longer necessary).

Answer the following questions to identify what to incorporate into your organization's policy:

- What new diagnostic tests, treatments, or other factors are developed that require staff members to add to their knowledge and expertise?
- What current competencies no longer meet the criteria for ongoing competency assessment? Are the treatments outdated, are they no longer initiated, or have they become part of a daily routine with reduced impact on patient outcome and little or no exceptional level of skill?
- What level of skill do new initiatives require?
- Who is authorized to perform/evaluate the effectiveness of new initiatives?
- What safety risks (to patients, visitors, and staff members) are associated with these new initiatives?
- How often will these new initiatives be implemented?

Think about your answer to the last question carefully. Staff members cannot achieve or retain competency unless they have fairly regular opportunities to use new knowledge and skills. Consider the following example:

A newly opened, freestanding 100-bed rehabilitation facility does not have 24-hour physician coverage on-site. The patient population consists primarily of spinal cord injury, stroke, traumatic head injury, hip fracture, multiple fracture, and amputee patients. Although the patients are relatively stable prior to their transfer to the facility, occasionally a patient deteriorates rapidly and emergency medical services (EMS) is notified. Patients also go into cardiac arrest. All direct patient care providers are CPR-certified. In the event of cardiac arrest, CPR is initiated and an IV is started, and the use of a portable defibrillator is sanctioned if warranted. This procedure was developed with the assistance of EMS personnel. The arrival of the EMS squad from the local acute-care health system takes between seven and 10 minutes.

The administrative staff (CEO, director of nursing, and comptroller) expressed concern that patients could not be intubated and advance life support drugs administered prior to the arrival of the EMS squad. They decided to mandate that all RNs working at the rehabilitation facility achieve and maintain advanced cardiac life support (ACLS) certification. These nurses, on the rare occasion of a cardiac arrest, would be expected to intubate patients and initiate ACLS treatment measures, including the administration of cardiac medications. The RNs would need to demonstrate ongoing competency in ACLS to keep their jobs. Is this a realistic competency?

The answer, of course, is no. Nurses cannot maintain competency in a procedure as complex as ACLS when they do not have regular opportunities to use such knowledge and skills. In fact, attempting to intubate a patient when you have an opportunity to do so only once a year is extremely dangerous.

The EMS representatives teamed up with the facility's staff development specialists to convince the administrative staff that attempting to mandate ACLS certification would do more harm than good. But until this was accomplished, the nursing staff was quite upset, and some even resigned rather than attempt to achieve ACLS certification.

This example illustrates the importance of being able to use knowledge and apply skills to achieve and maintain competency. Knowledge acquisition alone is not enough.

The checklist in Figure 5.1 may help you to document your assessment of the need for new competency development.

Figure 5.1

New competency assessment checklist

Date: ____________________

Item being evaluated:

- ❑ New equipment
- ❑ New treatment
- ❑ New medication
- ❑ New patient population
- ❑ Interpersonal communication issue
- ❑ Research initiatives

Identify the item specifically (e.g., type and purpose of equipment, description of new treatment, etc.).

1. What new knowledge/skills are required to safely initiate this new item?

2. Who is authorized to perform these new skills (e.g., RNs, LPNs, etc.)

3. What, if any, quality improvement/risk management data indicate a need for this competency?

4. What risks to patients, visitors, and staff members are associated with the new initiative?

5. How often will staff members have an opportunity to apply the new knowledge and skills necessary for safe, accurate implementation of this new initiative?

Figure 5.1

New competency assessment checklist (cont.)

There is a need for new competency development. The new competency is:

____

____

____

____

Signature, title, and date

There is no need for new competency development. The rationale for this is:

____

____

____

____

Signature, title, and date

Best practices for the implementation of new competencies

Unfortunately, new competencies do not evolve neatly on an annual basis, allowing ample time for appropriate education and training to occur. They pop up at any time, with varying degrees of urgency. Here are some suggestions for implementing new competencies (Cooper 2002).

Competency skills fairs

Some organizations have implemented day-long or half-day competency assessment days. These are called by various names, such as "skills fairs," "competency days," "competency skills labs," and so on. The premise is generally the same: A variety of competencies are assessed during a specified period and at an identified general location (usually a classroom setting). These events can be held at specified times throughout the year, such as annually, semiannually, or quarterly.

Advantages of this approach include the following:

- **Efficiency:** Competency days allow you to address the maximum number of people with a minimum number of observers.
- **Regular scheduling:** Staff members know when these events will occur and, in conjunction with their managers, can plan their attendance. Likewise, those responsible for organizing the competency days have planning time and the chance to add/delete competencies.
- **Decreased time away from the actual work site:** By planning regular assessment days, staffing needs can be planned in advance.

Disadvantages of this approach include the following:

- Competencies are added or deleted only at specific times throughout the year. This may compromise the timeliness of critical competency assessments.
- Competencies that require demonstration of actual patient-care interactions/procedures are not suitable for this approach.
- Having sufficient competency assessors on hand can be problematic.
- The length of time the fair is open can be a challenge. Twenty-four-hour availability requires a large number of competency assessors. If 24-hour availability is not possible, determining the hours of opera-

tion can draw complaints from staff members who must attend on their off time. In addition, because competency assessment is a mandate, staff members are entitled to be paid for attending these types of events, which can place a considerable burden on the organization's budget.

Drills and simulations

An evaluation form must be completed after each drill. This form serves as a record of behavior, a competency assessment, and a format to document strengths and areas for improvement. Examples of drills and simulations include mock codes, internal and external disasters, and hazardous-spill cleanup.

Drills and simulations:

- Require little or no additional staffing
- Can serve as a complement to the annual review of the environment of care plans required by the Occupational Safety & Health Administration
- Evaluate behavior in true-to-life situations

Disadvantages of drills and simulations are that they:

- May disrupt other programs or patient-care activities
- Require exceptionally well-qualified evaluators
- Need specific identification of required behaviors on evaluation forms

Performance improvement monitors

This approach relies on data from performance improvement (PI) documentation. PI indicators are useful when evaluating both interpersonal competencies and abilities to perform clinical skills.

Advantages of using PI monitors include the following:

- PI monitors are regular, reliable sources of data
- No additional time burden is required to collect the data
- Managers can simultaneously validate competency and complete a mandated activity without additional work, making the process more efficient

Disadvantages of using PI monitors include the following:

- They require the assumption that the PI data is accurate and objective
- They do not guarantee that competency was consistently evaluated if multiple people had input into the performance evaluation

Return demonstration/observation

Return demonstration can take place during the previously mentioned skills fair or on the job, which involves direct observation of skill performance.

Return demonstration/observation:

- Allows the assessor to actually see behavior and the employee's application of knowledge
- Allows for demonstration of new knowledge and skills in the actual work environment in "real-life" settings

Disadvantages of return demonstration/observation include the following:

- It may influence the behavior of the staff member being assessed because he or she is aware that an evaluation is taking place
- It cannot guarantee that employees' behavior is the same during the return demonstration/observation as when not being observed

Self-assessment

Self-assessment generally requires that employees complete a written exercise designed to identify their beliefs and knowledge about their job performance. The employees' assessment is compared to the managers' and other assessors' assessments. Any disparity must be addressed so that job performance improves.

Self-assessment:

- Helps employees to recognize their own beliefs and values and how these issues may affect their job performance
- Identifies incongruence between employees' beliefs and values and the organization's mission, vision, and values

Disadvantages of self-assessment include the following:

- It does not provide an opportunity for evaluation of the actual behaviors
- Results are influenced by employees' and assessors' personal values and beliefs
- Failure to address incongruence results in employees continuing to behave in ways that are inconsistent with the organization's mission, vision, and values

Dimensions of competencies

Each approach is distinct and focuses on specific aspects of employee skills. According to *Competency Assessment: A Practical Guide to the JCAHO Standards, 2nd edition* (Summers et al 2004), competencies are designed to evaluate particular features of skills, called *dimensions*. Each dimension includes explicit skills and knowledge. They include the following:

- *Critical-thinking dimension: the ability to use information or knowledge, including:*
  - Problem-solving
  - Planning
  - Clinical reasoning
  - Adapting to/facilitating change
  - Time management
  - Fiscal responsibility

- *Interpersonal dimension: the ability to work effectively with others, including:*
  - Communication
  - Conflict management
  - Customer service
  - Working effectively with members of various cultures and racial and ethnic backgrounds
  - Working as effective team players

- *Technical dimension: the possession of knowledge and the ability to use that knowledge to perform fine and gross motor functions, including:*
  - Cognitive abilities
  - Acquired knowledge
  - Psychomotor ability
  - Technical competence

As you evaluate the need for new competencies, review these dimensions to determine both need and approach. Remember that a competency assessment program focuses on verifying and validating skills and knowledge application in the workplace. The purpose of a competency program is to:

- Improve job performance
- Enhance patient outcomes
- Promote economic efficiency
- Increase organizational effectiveness

Demonstrated achievement of these goals shows that your competency assessment program is one that not only validates knowledge and skills, but also results in improved patient outcomes.

REFERENCES

1. Avillion A. 2004. *A Practical Guide to Staff Development: Tools and Techniques for Effective Education*. Marblehead, MA: HCPro, Inc.

2. Cooper, D. 2002. "The 'C' Word: Competency" in Kristen L. O'Shea, *Staff Development Nursing Secrets*. Philadelphia: Hanley & Belfus.

3. Summers, B., Tracy, J., and Woods, W. 2004. *Competency Assessment: A Practical Guide to the JCAHO Standards, 2nd Edition*. Marblehead, MA: HCPro, Inc..

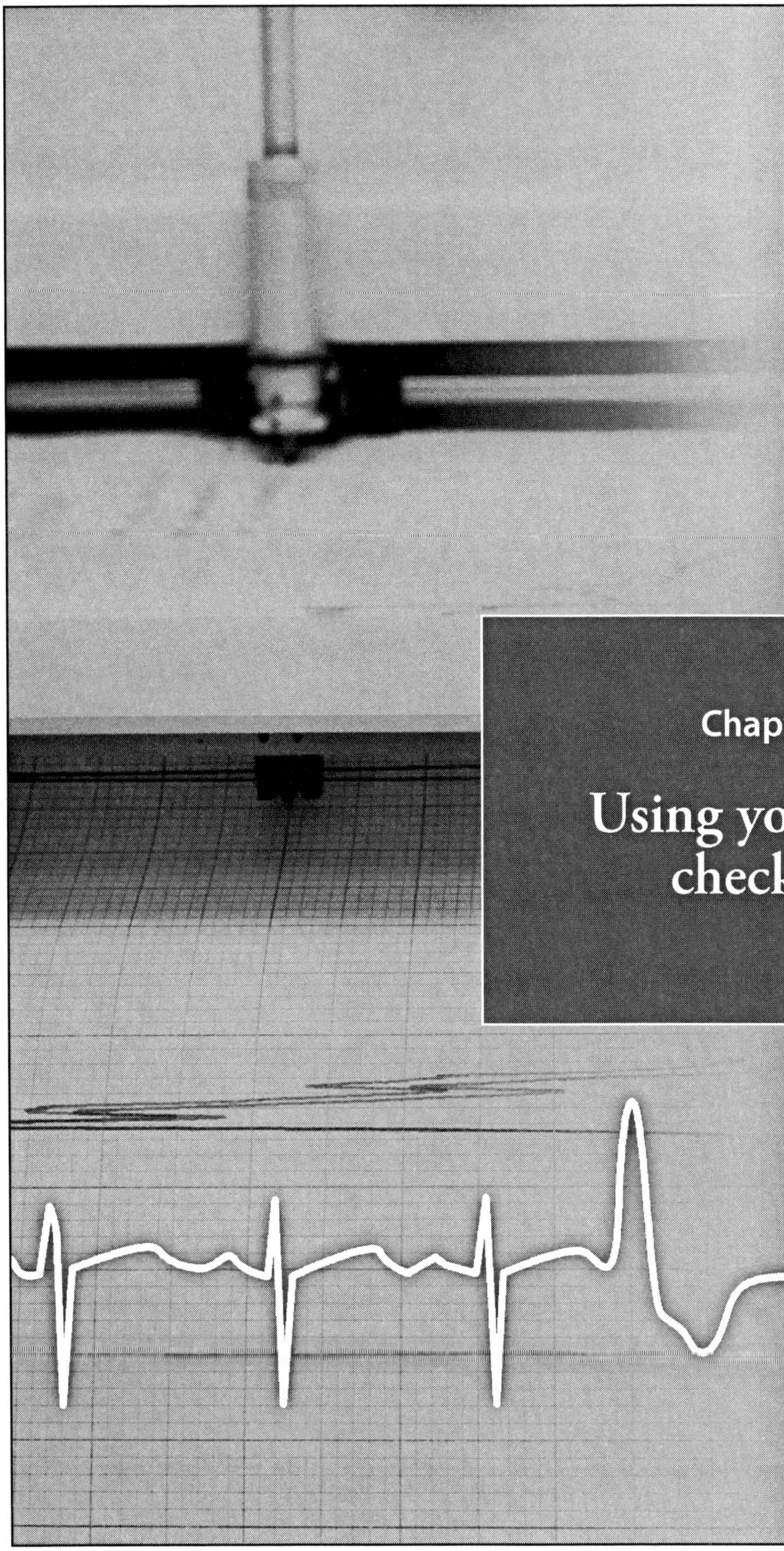

Chapter 6

Using your skills checklists

Chapter 6

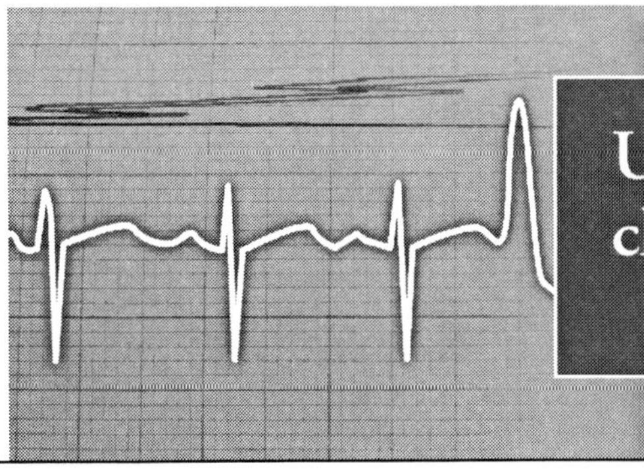

Using your skills checklists

Learning objectives

After reading this chapter, the participant should be able to:

- Differentiate between difference between orientation checklists and skills checklists

Skills checklists must clearly identify expectations and should be completed by staff members who know how to use them. Criteria for safe, effective performance must be clearly defined, and everyone participating in the evaluation process must have a common understanding of the criteria and the basis for assigning ratings. Research has shown that if evaluators make direct observations using precise measurement criteria in checklists, with immediate feedback on performance, this is more effective than the traditional evaluation of clinical skills using subjective rating forms. The format for skills checklists may vary, but most contain similar information. Regardless of how they are used, skills checklists should:

- Be learner-oriented
- Focus on behaviors
- Be measurable
- Use criteria validated by experts
- Be specific enough to avoid ambiguity

A template used to create the skills checklists included in this manual appears in Figure 6.1, and an electronic version of this template appears on your accompanying CD-ROM; you can open it as a Microsoft Word document. The individual's name and date are important to identify whose skills are being validated and when the evaluation is being conducted.

Figure 6.1

Skills checklist template

Name: ______________________________ Date: ____________________

Skill:

Steps	Completed	Comments

Self-assessment	Evaluation/ validation methods	Levels	Type of validation	Comments
❑ Experienced ❑ Need practice ❑ Never done ❑ Not applicable (based on scope of practice)	❑ Verbal ❑ Demonstration/ observation ❑ Practical exercise ❑ Interactive class	❑ Beginner ❑ Intermediate ❑ Expert	❑ Orientation ❑ Annual ❑ Other _____	

______________________________ ______________________________

Employee signature *Observer signature*

The steps identified in the checklist should define the critical behaviors needed for effective performance of the skill and do not include every step of the procedure. You can use the "Completed" column to indicate that each step was performed correctly, but note that some checklists use a met/not met format instead. It is helpful if checklists include an area for comments. Also note that most checklists are used to evaluate a single occurrence.

In the checklist format just described, the self-assessment can give the evaluator an idea of the individual's perceived skill level, although that can never take the place of validating competency. Individuals may have different perceptions of their abilities that may or may not be consistent with the evaluator's perceptions. For instance, one person could indicate that he or she needs practice, even though that person is familiar and competent with that skill but is not familiar with the institution's policy and procedure. Another staff member could indicate that he or she needs practice because the staff member has performed the skill only once during his or her career. All required skills must be validated, regardless of the individual's assessment of his or her ability.

The evaluation/validation method areas indicate how the validation was performed. The method used most often is demonstration or observation of the individual performing the skill, but verbal questioning can also be effective in identifying the thought processes or critical thinking involved with skills. Practical exercises and interactive class activities can also be useful as validation methods.

The appropriate level (beginner, intermediate, or expert) can be indicated, as well as the type of validation. It is important to identify whether the assessment is part of an individual's orientation or whether it is an ongoing annual validation. It is also important that you have both the employee and the observer sign the checklist.

The Joint Commission mandates that all employees have their competence assessed upon hire and throughout their employment. One way to meet this standard is to have orientation checklists in addition to skills checklists (Joint Commission Resources 2008).

Differences between orientation checklists and skills checklists

Orientation checklists specify the knowledge, attitudes, and skills needed to perform safely. The information for an orientation checklist would come from the position description for that job classification and would outline the essential competencies for safe practice in that role. Skills checklists, on the other hand, include the specific tasks related to a policy or procedure. Skills checklists are often used to document ongoing competency, as compared to orientation checklists, which document initial competency.

Developing orientation checklists

Key elements in developing an orientation checklist are the job description and performance evaluation criteria. The components of the orientation program provide the framework. Essential information in the checklist would include the individual's name and the names of all evaluators. The hire date and unit are helpful to identify when the individual started in his or her role. Orientation checklists provide documentation of the initial assessment of competence required by The Joint Commission, as well as the individual's self-assessment. If evaluation during the orientation is a shared responsibility (e.g., with staff development educators and unit preceptors), different columns can be used to identify what was done during a classroom orientation and what was done in the clinical area. A "Not Evaluated" or "Not Applicable" column can be helpful for those skills that an orientee did not have an opportunity to perform during the orientation process.

Sample checklists for RN orientation (Figure 6.2) and nursing assistant (NA) orientation (Figure 6.3) are included as examples.

Orientation checklists should be developed with input from the management staff. This will ensure that they include the essential skills expected from the position. Generally, staff development personnel/preceptors complete orientation checklists. Preceptors help new employees adjust to the workplace and clinical unit, and they work with new employees to help plan the learning experiences and share knowledge of expected behaviors. They can help to reduce stress and enhance learning for new employees by using adult learning principles, documenting skill acquisition, and helping the new person socialize into the unit culture. The checklist helps to make employees accountable for their learning by clearly identifying expectations to be completed during the orientation period. After the orientation checklist is completed, it usually becomes part of the employee's permanent file, which protects both the employer and the employee.

Figure 6.2

Competency-based orientation checklist

SUMMA HEALTH SYSTEM STAFF DEVELOPMENT
RN SKILLS ASSESSMENT/EVALUATION

NAME: ________________________ **HIRE DATE:** ________________________
UNIT: ____

STAFF DEVELOPMENT:	INITIALS:	PRECEPTORS:	INITIALS:
____________	______	____________	______
____________	______	____________	______
____________	______	____________	______
____________	______		
____________	______		

Directions:

Orientee: Complete the self-assessment by placing a check (✓) in the appropriate column based on your level of familiarity or experience with each competency.

Staff Development/Preceptor: Complete the evaluation section for each competency after the orientee has demonstrated successful completion of that competency. Place the date and your initials in the appropriate column. If NE (not evaluated) is checked, include an explanation in the comments column.

	SELF-ASSESSMENT			EVALUATION			
Competencies	Comfortable	Need Review	Have never done	* SD ORT	Unit	**NE	Comments
I. Competency A. Applies a systematic problem-solving approach in the implementation of nursing plans of care:							
1. Uses nursing process to systematically assess, plan, implement and evaluate nursing care.							

***SD ORT = Staff Development Orientation **NE = If Not Evaluated, indicate explanation**

Figure 6.2

Competency-based orientation checklist (cont.)

2. Provide/documents patient teaching/ discharge planning.						
3. Involves patient/ significant other in plan of care .						
4. Prioritizes nursing care for a group of patients.						
5. Initiates patient referrals as needed.						
6. Utilizes appropriate resources.						
B. Intravenous therapy 1. Initiates intravenous						
2. Monitors intravenous according to policy and procedure a. Checks rate						
b. Assesses for signs and symptoms of complications						
c. Initiates PRN adapter						
3. Uses infusion pumps correctly: • PCA						
• Baxter						
4. Draws blood specimens: • Routine						
• Central line						
• Blood cultures						
5. Administers blood and blood components.						

***SD ORT = Staff Development Orientation **NE = If Not Evaluated, indicate explanation**

Figure 6.2

Competency-based orientation checklist (cont.)

6. Maintains central line/ hyperalimentation.							
7. Applies/changes central line dressing.							
8. Administers IV medications (I.V.P.B. IV push).							
9. Documents administration of IV Therapy.							
10. Completes IV Therapy exam with a minimum score of 80%							
C. Medication administration 1. Describes usual dose, common side effects, compatibilities, action, and untoward reactions of medications.							
2. Administers medications							
a. I.M.							
b. SQ and Insulin							
c. Calculations							
d. Other							
3. Documents administration of medications (MAR, controlled drugs, etc.).							
4. Identifies medication error reporting system.							
D. Treatment and procedures 1. Inserts and maintains gastric feeding tubes.							

***SD ORT = Staff Development Orientation **NE = If Not Evaluated, indicate explanation**

Figure 6.2

Competency-based orientation checklist (cont.)

2. Inserts and maintains urinary catheters.							
3. Performs trach care and suctioning.							
4. Assesses patient safety including proper utilization of restraints.							
5. Completes tissue therapy SLP.							
6. Provides and documents pre-and postop nursing care.							
7. Incorporates nursing measures to reduce and prevent the spread of infection in daily nursing care.							
8. Completes American Heart Association guidelines for BLS-C in CPR.							
9. Changes oxygen gauge and sets rate.							
10. Locates various items on the emergency cart.							
11. Identifies nursing responsibilities in emergency situations.							
12. Completes: a. Admission of patient							
b. Transfer of a patient							
c. Discharge of a patient							
13. Performs neurological checks when appropriate.							

***SD ORT = Staff Development Orientation **NE = If Not Evaluated, indicate explanation**

Figure 6.2

Competency-based orientation checklist (cont.)

14. Performs BGT.							
15. Other.							
II. Communication A. Documents on the following forms: • Initial Interdisciplinary Assessment							
• Graphic Record							
• Interdisciplinary Progress Record							
• Nursing Discharge/ Patient Teaching							
• Interdisciplinary Plan of Care							
• Unusual Occurrence							
B. Transcribes physician's orders.							
C. Takes verbal orders from physician.							
D. Uses correct lines of communication.							
E. Attends Computer Class							
F. Gives prompt, accurate, and pertinent shift report.							
G. Interacts with patients significant others and health team members in positive manner.							

***SD ORT = Staff Development Orientation **NE = If Not Evaluated, indicate explanation**

Figure 6.2

Competency-based orientation checklist (cont.)

III. Accountability/Leadership A. Completes orientation statement of agreement.							
B. Delegates patient care to other personnel appropriately.							
C. Follows appropriate employee policies and procedures, i.e. call off, time off, LOA, etc.							
D. Conforms to dress code.							
E. Identifies role of the nurse in quality assurance.							
F. Maintains safe working environment.							
G. Contains costs through proper use of supplies and maintenance of equipment.							
IV. Other A. Has completed Human Resource/Safety Orientation							

***SD ORT = Staff Development Orientation **NE = If Not Evaluated, indicate explanation**

Figure 6.2

Competency-based orientation checklist (cont.)

RELEASE FROM ORIENTATION

The undersigned employee/orientee can be released from orientation as of ________________ (date).

____________________	____________________	____________________
Orientee Signature	Preceptor Signature	Unit Manager Signature

Return this form and orientation paperwork/folder to ACH Nursing Records or STH Human Resources when completed.

Skills still needing supervision are listed below. It is the responsibility of the employee/orientee to be supervised prior to performing these skills: ____

____

____

***SD ORT = Staff Development Orientation **NE = If Not Evaluated, indicate explanation**

Source: Summa Health System Hospitals, Akron, OH. Reprinted with permission.

Figure 6.3

Nursing assistant orientation checklist

SUMMA HEALTH SYSTEM HOSPITALS
STAFF DEVELOPMENT

COMPETENCY-BASED CHECKLIST

NURSING ASSISTANT ORIENTATION
SKILLS ASSESSMENT/EVALUATION

NAME: ____________________
HIRE DATE (this role): ____________
UNIT: ____________________

STAFF DEVELOPMENT:	INITIALS:	PRECEPTORS:	INITIALS:
____________	________	____________	______
____________	________	____________	______
____________	________	____________	______

Directions:

Orientee: Complete the self-assessment by placing a check (✓) in the appropriate column based on your level of familiarity or experience with each competency.

Staff Development/Preceptor: Complete the evaluation section for each competency after the orientee has demonstrated successful completion of that competency. Place the date and your initials in the appropriate column. If NE (not evaluated) is checked, include an explanation in the comments column.

	SELF-ASSESSMENT			EVALUATION			
Competencies	Comfortable	Need Review	Have never done	* SD ORT	Unit	**NE	Comments
A. Demonstrates ability to do basic patient care as follows: 1. Complete bed bath							
2. Partial bath							
3. Assists with shower							
4. Oral hygiene							

***SD ORT = Staff Development Orientation **NE = If Not Evaluated, indicate explanation**

Figure 6.3

Nursing assistant orientation checklist (cont.)

5. Back care							
6. Peri care							
7. Hair care							
8. Offering/removal of bed pan/urinal							
9. Cath care							
10. Documentation of output on Kardex or worksheet							Unit based competency on file.
11. Feeding of patient, including compensatory strategies for feeding dysphagic patient							
12. Shaving of patient							
13. Occupied bed							
14. Unoccupied bed							
15. Accurately measuring patient intake and output and recording on appropriate form							
16. Patient transfer/ discharge							
17. Pneumatic Cuffs							
18. K-Pad							
B. Body mechanics 1. Discusses the proper techniques of lifting/ turning/transferring patient							
2. Demonstrates proper technique in transferring patient from bed to cart and back							

***SD ORT = Staff Development Orientation **NE = If Not Evaluated, indicate explanation**

Figure 6.3

Nursing assistant orientation checklist (cont.)

3. Demonstrates proper technique transferring patient from bed to wheelchair							
4. Demonstrates proper technique in positioning and turning patients							
C. Technical skills 1. Assesses patient safety including proper utilization and documentation of restraints							
2. Completes American Heart Association guidelines for Heartsaver Course							
3. Monitors oxygen tank gauge							
4. Identifies responsibilities in emergency situations							
5. Incorporates measures to reduce and prevent the spread of infection in daily patient care							
D. Demonstrates ability to take and record vital signs. Temperature: 1. Takes oral temperature and records 2. Discusses procedure for rectal temperature							Unit based competency checklist on file.

***SD ORT = Staff Development Orientation **NE = If Not Evaluated, indicate explanation**

Figure 6.3

Nursing assistant orientation checklist (cont.)

Radial pulse: 1. Counts and records pulse rate							
Respirations: 1. Counts respiratory rate and records							
E. Demonstrates ability to obtain and transport appropriately the following specimens: 1. Sputum							
2. Urine/routine/ccms							
3. Stool							
4. Blood, transport only							
F. Performs postmortem care							
G. Transports patient to morgue							
H. Removes dirty linen or equipment from patient room							
I. Passes and picks up trays							
1. Records intake (and output) accurately on worksheet in room.							Unit based competency checklist on file.
2. Empty and replace trash bags, remove excess linen, etc., from patient rooms							

***SD ORT = Staff Development Orientation **NE = If Not Evaluated, indicate explanation**

Figure 6.3

Nursing assistant orientation checklist (cont.)

K. Maintenance needs 1. Verbalizes safety issues with equipment (step ladders, hand tools, light bulbs, etc.)						
2. Identifies light maintenance duties						
L. Demonstrates ability to Assess Just-In-Time technician. (Distribution)						
M. Demonstrates proper use of communication 1. Patient intercom						Unit based competency checklist on file.
2. Answering patient call light						
3. Telephone/answering phone appropriately by identifying unit, name, and status						
4. Operating pneumatic tube system, describe purpose and use						
5. Explaining the importance of patient confidentiality						
6. Communicating to RN any unusual observations (signs and symptoms)						
N. Interacts with patients, significant others, and health team members in positive manner.						

***SD ORT = Staff Development Orientation **NE = If Not Evaluated, indicate explanation**

Figure 6.3

Nursing assistant orientation checklist (cont.)

O. Safety issues (Each orientee should be able to discuss and correctly answer questions on the following safety topics) 1. Fire safety (Code Red)							
2. Bomb threat (Code Black)							
3. Code violet							
4. Infection prevention and exposure control							
5. Disaster (Code yellow)							
6. Evacuation							
7. Back safety							
8. Severe weather							
9. Electrical safety							
10. Code Adam							
P. Punctuality 1. Arrives on unit in uniform on time							
2. Notifies nursing office of absence according to policy							
3. Notifies nursing office of lateness according to policy							
4. Notifies nurse in charge when leaving unit and reason							

***SD ORT = Staff Development Orientation **NE = If Not Evaluated, indicate explanation**

Figure 6.3

Nursing assistant orientation checklist (cont.)

5. Follows current hospital guidelines for breaks and lunch hours							
6. Returns from errands and meetings promptly							
Q. Examinations Completes the following exams with a minimum score of 70%: 1. Medical Abbreviation Test							
2. Patient Safety Test							
3. Patient Limited Activity Test							
4. Grooming and Oral Hygiene Test							
R. Other:							

***SD ORT = Staff Development Orientation **NE = If Not Evaluated, indicate explanation**

Source: Summa Health System Hospitals, Akron, OH. Reprinted with permission.

Skills checklists for annual competency assessment

This section provides suggestions on how to determine what skills to evaluate, develop the skills checklists, identify who can complete the checklists, and keep track of who has been evaluated. It also reviews what happens if someone does not meet identified competencies, and it includes a brief discussion of other methods of validating competence.

Determining what skills to evaluate

Your organization needs to set up a system to determine which competencies to evaluate each year. Chapter 2 provided a suggested formula to use when determining which skills to evaluate. There is no right or wrong way to select what skills will be evaluated, as long as the organization can justify why the particular skills were chosen. Skills should be selected based on the individual needs of the unit or organization.

Developing the skills checklists

Once the skills to be assessed are selected, skills checklists can be developed or modified from the samples attached to ensure consistency in evaluation. Review your institution's policies and procedures using current literature for support. The essential steps of the policies and procedures are incorporated into the skills checklists, many of which you can easily adapt for your institution by changing the criteria to be consistent with steps in your policies and procedures or standards.

Identifying who can complete the checklists

It is important to identify who (e.g., what job classification) can validate skills for each job classification. It may be better to have an RN or licensed practical nurse check off an NA on vital signs rather than to have another NA complete the skills checklist. Individuals who are responsible for validating someone's skill should be qualified based on education, experience, or expertise with that skill, or they should have already demonstrated proficiency with that skill. An individual with documented competence in that skill should assess ongoing competence. That competence may be determined by his or her role (e.g., advanced practice nurse, staff development instructor, unit managers, specialist coordinator, etc.), frequency of performing the skill, or already having demonstrated competence in that skill.

When introducing new technology or procedures into the clinical area, the initial training should be done by individuals with documented experience in that procedure (e.g., physicians, nurses from that specialty, vendor representatives, etc.). A core group of staff members or a single individual can be trained and can confirm the competency of other staff members after they personally demonstrate competence in that skill.

Keeping track of who has been evaluated

Each evaluator should refer to the skills checklist when observing a staff member perform that skill. Skills checklists for the competencies being evaluated can be kept in a competency notebook as a reference for the staff. These checklists can be used to assess initial and ongoing competence. The use of a checklist ensures consistency in evaluating the steps to perform the skill. Rather than completing an individual skills checklist for every person evaluated, a tracking sheet can usually be used to document completion of that skill.

The tracking sheet provides a way to document that staff members in each classification have completed required competencies. Names of the unit personnel are written on the tracking sheet, and when someone is checked off on a particular competency, the individual observing that person writes in the date and his or her initials in the column for that particular competency in the row with that person's name. Individuals are responsible for ensuring that someone validates their required skills each year. The manager then uses this information when completing performance appraisals.

The Competencies Analyzer

Figure 6.4 provides a sample tracking sheet. We've also provided an electronic version of this Excel spreadsheet on your accompanying CD-ROM. The Competencies Analyzer is an easy way for a manager to track competency assessment on his or her unit.

Figure 6.4

Competencies tracking sheet

SUMMA HEALTH SYSTEM HOSPITALS
UNIT BASED COMPETENCY CHECKLIST
Unit Secretary

MEDICAL SURGICAL UNIT: ____________________

EMPLOYEE NAME	COMPETENCY VERIFIED								
	SUMMA	DEPT	DIVISION	UNIT BASED					
	1. Mandatory Safety Education	2. Heart Saver	See schedule for Mandatory Ed. and SLPs						

Source: Summa Health System Hospitals, Akron, OH. Reprinted with permission.

Determining what happens when a staff member cannot perform competencies

Organizations need to identify the consequences when a staff member cannot demonstrate mastery of a competency. Policies may vary, but a mechanism needs to be in place to safeguard patients and ensure that the staff member is not assigned to a patient who requires that competency. Possible options would be to provide remediation and further clinical experiences, or to transfer the staff member to another area where he or she can meet the required competencies. Continued failure to demonstrate required competencies may lead to a plan for improvement or termination.

Other methods to validate competence

It is also important to realize that the skills checklists are only one method to validate competence; other methods may be used. Some skills may not happen frequently enough to check all staff members off on that skill, and skills fairs may be an alternative approach. During skills fairs, employees are tested and validated on skills using simulations, games, word puzzles, or other methods to verify that they are aware of the steps of the procedure. Skills checklists can also be used during fairs for those skills that may not come up frequently enough to check everyone on a unit.

With the increasing sophistication of technology, computer-assisted video evaluation may be used to evaluate competency in a particular area. Videotaped or simulated scenarios can give evaluators the opportunity to observe and rate performances. With this approach, ratings can be compared with the instructor to clarify any discrepancies and determine inter-rater reliability. However, this may not be realistic in organizations where many staff members will be completing skills checklists for their peers.

One problem with skills checklists is that you don't know whether the observed behavior is persistent and representative of the situation being observed, or whether the individual is going through the correct steps knowing that someone is evaluating him or her for that single occurrence. Therefore, indirect observation can also be used. Often, managers or charge nurses conduct patient rounds and medical record reviews. With indirect observation, there may not be direct observation of the skills, but there is the presumption that the skills are correctly followed when the desired outcomes are achieved. Clinical rounds can measure competencies as well as improve the standard of care and practice in the clinical setting.

Organizations need to have a competency-based program in place to ensure that individuals are prepared to deliver quality patient care. Assessment of competency begins with orientation and continues throughout employment. An evaluation of each nursing staff member's competency should be conducted at defined intervals throughout the individual's association with the organization. Performance appraisals and skills checklists may be used to measure the ongoing competency of nursing employees. Continuing education programs and inservices can also enhance staff members' competency.

Competence assessment for the nursing staff and volunteers who provide direct patient care is based on the following:

- Populations served, including age ranges and specialties
- Competencies required for role and provision of care
- Competencies assessed during orientation
- Unit-specific competencies that need to be assessed or reassessed on a yearly basis based on care modalities, age ranges, techniques, procedures, technology, equipment, skills needed, or changes in laws and regulations
- Appropriate assessment methods for the skill being assessed
- Delineation of who is qualified to assess competence
- A description of action taken when improvement activities lead to a determination that a staff member with performance problems is unable or unwilling to improve

Individuals who transfer from another area in the organization know what competencies they must meet at the time of their orientation.

Here is a list of some questions to consider in an evaluation of the competence assessment system (Cooper 2002):

- Is new-employee competence assessment completed during the initial orientation process?
- Is employee orientation based on assessed competencies and the knowledge and skills required to deliver patient-care services?

- Is new-employee competence assessment completed at the conclusion of the orientation process?
- Do clinical staff members participate in ongoing educational activities to acquire new competencies that support patient-care delivery? Are those activities minimally based on quality improvement findings, new technology, therapeutic or pharmacology interventions, and the learning needs of the nursing staff?
- Does the management or leadership staff participate in competence assessment activities (i.e., clinical knowledge, skills, or technology)?
- Does the management or leadership staff participate in ongoing education activities to acquire new competencies for patient-care management (i.e., management development)?
- Does the performance evaluation system address staff competence?
- When competency deficiencies are noted, is a plan for correction initiated and implemented?
- Does reassessment of competence occur as necessary?
- Are summaries of competence assessment findings available by individual, by patient-care unit, and by department?
- Are plans for competence maintenance and improvement documented?
- Is an annual report submitted to the governing body?
- Do policies and procedures exist to define the process of competence assessment?

The overall competence assessment process must be reviewed on an ongoing basis to determine its effectiveness and any opportunities for improvement. This evaluation identifies what works, what doesn't, why it doesn't, and how it can be improved. It can take a very formal approach through survey methodology and interviews, or a less formal approach of asking for subjective data and feedback from key people and groups.

REFERENCES

1. Joint Commission Resources. (2008). *Comprehensive Accreditation Manual for Hospitals: The Official Handbook*. Oakbrook, IL: Joint Commission Resources.

2. Cooper, D. (2002). "The 'C' Word: Competency" in Kristen L. O'Shea, *Staff Development Nursing Secrets*. Philadelphia: Hanley & Belfus.

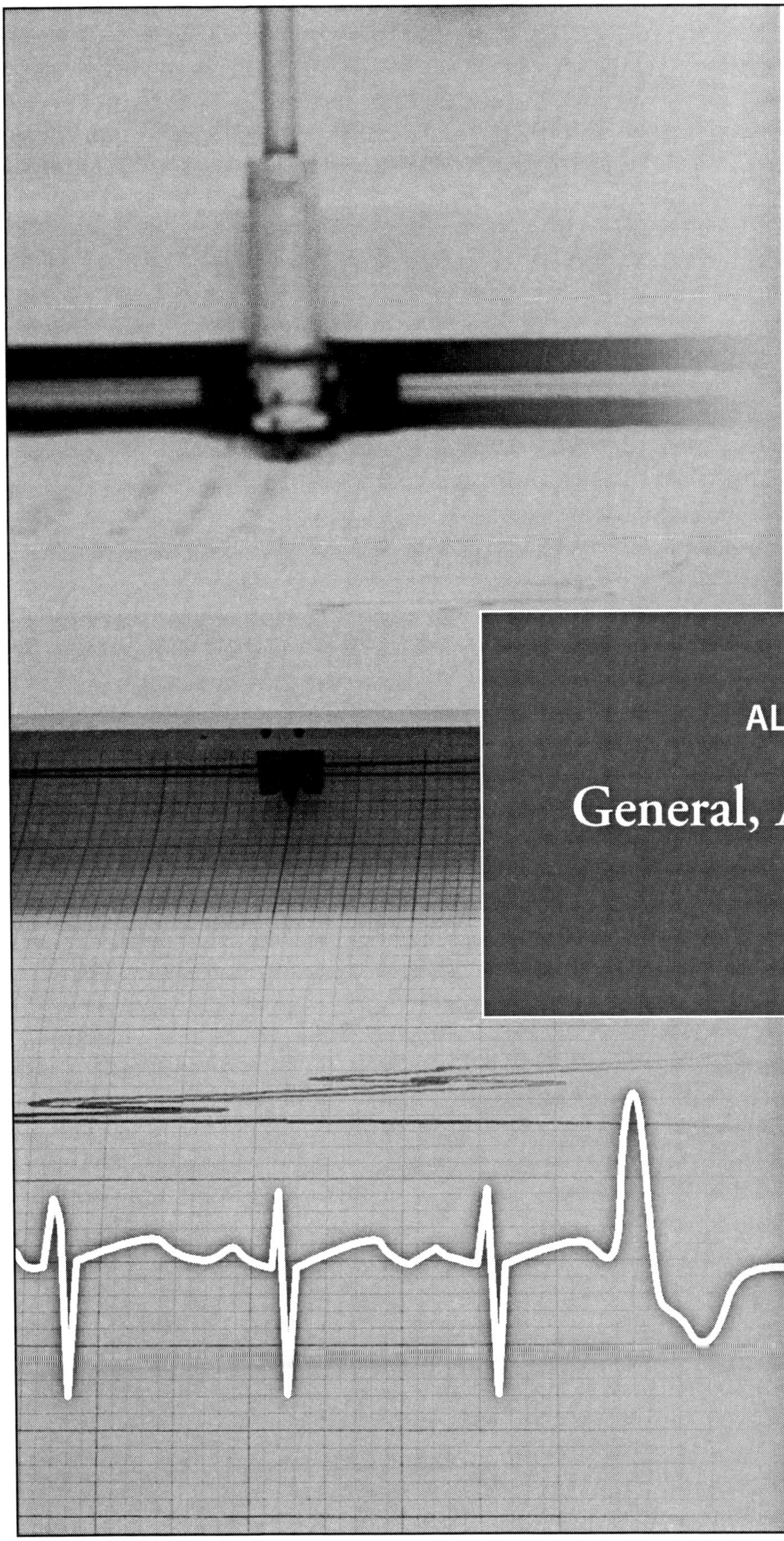

ALL

General, All Units

Contents

Name: ______________________________ Date: ______________

Skill: **ABG Interpretation**

Steps	Completed	Comments
1. Verbalizes normal ABG values pH pCO_2 pO_2 HCO_3		
2. Using available assessment and laboratory data, accurately determines patient's acid/base status. • Normal • Respiratory Acidosis • Respiratory Alkalosis • Metabolic Acidosis • Metabolic Alkalosis • Mixed Respiratory/Metabolic Acidosis or • Alkalosis		
3. Identifies at least one physical sign and/or symptom associated with the patient's ABG interpretation.		
4. Identifies at least one intervention to assist the patient in returning to a normal acid/base bal-ance.		
5. Makes appropriate referral to physician or respiratory therapist as indicated by AFB findings.		

Self-assessment	Evaluation/ validation methods	Levels	Type of validation	Comments
❑ Experienced ❑ Need practice ❑ Never done ❑ Not applicable (based on scope of practice)	❑ Verbal ❑ Demonstration/ observation ❑ Practical exercise ❑ Interactive class	❑ Beginner ❑ Intermediate ❑ Expert	❑ Orientation ❑ Annual ❑ Other _____	

______________________________ ______________________________

Employee signature *Observer signature*

Reference:

Urdern, LD: Stacy, KM and Lough, ME, eds (2006). Thelan's Critical Care Nursing: Diagnosis and Management, 5th Ed. Mosby Elsevier, St. Louis, MO. P604-606.

Name: ______________________________ Date: ______________

Skill: **Annual Competency Performance—Quality of Instruction**

Steps	Completed	Comments
1. Develops objectives that are relevant, realistic and measurable.		
2. Incorporates teaching/learning strategies to address identified needs and goals.		
3. Uses up-to-date accurate resources/materials in presentation.		
4. Picks up on verbal and nonverbal cues during session.		
5. Ensures any handouts are easily read, free of errors, and attractively designed.		
6. Bases audiovisuals on the size of the group, setting and equipment available.		
7. Provides pertinent information useful to practice.		

Self-assessment	Evaluation/ validation methods	Levels	Type of validation	Comments
❑ Experienced ❑ Need practice ❑ Never done ❑ Not applicable (based on scope of practice)	❑ Verbal ❑ Demonstration/ observation ❑ Practical exercise ❑ Interactive class	❑ Beginner ❑ Intermediate ❑ Expert	❑ Orientation ❑ Annual ❑ Other _____	

_______________________ _______________________

Employee signature ***Observer signature***

Reference:

Brunt, B. 2007. *Competencies for Staff Educators: Tools to Evaluate and Enhance Nursing Professional Development*. Marblehead, MA: HCPro, Inc.

Name: ____________________ Date: ____________

Skill: **Arjo Ceiling Lift**

Steps	Completed	Comments
1. Assures motor is in "charge" position when unit not in use.		
2. Identifies location and purpose of operational light indicator.		
3. Identifies red cord and explains its purpose.		
4. Uses handset to: a. Move lift motor off charger to desired position b. Lower and raise carry bar c. Move lift motor back to charger		
5. Demonstrates correct position of bed patient in sling and moves patient to chair a. Wraps sling legs properly b. Attaches sling loops to hook-up points on carry bar c. Stabilizes carry bar and patient while moving patient up and over to chair d. Lowers patient to chair e. Detaches sling from carry bar		
6. Returns unit to charge position using battery icon on handset.		
7. Locates manual operations wrench (Allen wrench) and its insertion point.		
8. Demonstrates manual operation of carry bar busing the Allen wrench.		
9. Verbalized how to clean cover of carry bar.		

Self-assessment	Evaluation/ validation methods	Levels	Type of validation	Comments
❑ Experienced ❑ Need practice ❑ Never done ❑ Not applicable (based on scope of practice)	❑ Verbal ❑ Demonstration/ observation ❑ Practical exercise ❑ Interactive class	❑ Beginner ❑ Intermediate ❑ Expert	❑ Orientation ❑ Annual ❑ Other _____	

____________________ ____________________

Employee signature ***Observer signature***

Reference:

Doloresco, L., Lloyd, T., Smith, L., and Weinel, D. 2002. A clinical evaluation of ceiling lifts: Lifting and transfer technology for the future. *SCI Nurse* 19(2): 75-77.

Name: ______________________________ Date: ______________

Skill: **Assessment/Validation of Competencies**

Steps	Completed	Comments
1. Demonstrates proficiency in skill being validated.		
2. Uses appropriate validation method(s).		
3. Validates performance according to established standards, e.g., checklist.		
4. Provides appropriate feedback to learner.		
5. Documents competency on appropriate form(s).		

Self-assessment	Evaluation/ validation methods	Levels	Type of validation	Comments
❑ Experienced ❑ Need practice ❑ Never done ❑ Not applicable (based on scope of practice)	❑ Verbal ❑ Demonstration/ observation ❑ Practical exercise ❑ Interactive class	❑ Beginner ❑ Intermediate ❑ Expert	❑ Orientation ❑ Annual ❑ Other _____	

______________________________ ______________________________

Employee signature ***Observer signature***

Reference:

Brunt, B. 2007. *Competencies for Staff Educators: Tools to Evaluate and Enhance Nursing Professional Development.* Marblehead, MA: HCPro, Inc.

Name: ______________________________ Date: ______________

Skill: **Assisting an Adult with Feeding**

Steps	Completed	Comments
1. Removes distasteful sights & odors from room, provides adequate ventilation, and clean surroundings for mealtime.		
2. Offers patient hand cleansing with a warm wash cloth & soap, or disinfecting gel.		
3. Positions patient comfortably upright in a chair, if possible. • Consults ST/RN/MD for best positioning of patient if unable to get into chair.		
4. Washes hands and brings tray to area.		
5. Verifies that the patient has the correct diet on tray, checks armband; asks patient to verify name, and doctor, or other identifying data.		
6. Ensures that diet is correct in PLATO, agrees with ST recommendations.		
7. Ensures food is the correct temperature and that liquids are thickened as ordered. Rewarms food and/or thickens liquids as needed.		
8. Prepares food, if necessary, by opening cartons, buttering bread, and cutting meat.		
9. Identifies foods, & describes location to patient.		
10. Drapes patient with towel or napkins.		
11. Sits in a comfortable position to feed the patient.		
12. Offers the patient small amounts of food at a time. Offers liquids as requested or between bites. • Follows speech therapist guidelines, i.e., positioning chin down towards chest when swallowing, or other positions to assist the patient as ordered.		
13. Lets the patient choose what he or she would like to eat next, unless directed by ST order.		
14. Warns patient about hot food and waits for it to cool.		
15. Does not rush the patient. Allows patient to chew and swallow the food before offering more. Uses a spoon to feed patient.		

• If new swallowing problems are observed, refers patient immediately for Bedside Swallow screening by RN, or ST per unit protocol.		
16. Encourages patient to hold bread or toast and to feed self when possible.		
17. Wipes the patient's mouth and chin when necessary.		
18. Allows for rest periods for the patient who tires easily.		
19. Moves the tray away from the patient.		
20. Checks the patient's gown and bed for spillage of food.		
21. Replaces any items removed from the bedside table (call light, telephone, urinal, Kleenex, etc.).		
22. Offers mouth care and hand washing after eating.		
23. Repositions the patient comfortably. • If at risk for aspiration, has the head of bed elevated for 30 minutes after eating and follows ST guidelines.		
24. Records fluids on I&O record on the door.		
25. Records percentage of meal eaten in patient record on PLATO.		
26. If patient on a calorie count, unit may collect Menus for calorie count in envelope on door.		

Self-assessment	Evaluation/ validation methods	Levels	Type of validation	Comments
❑ Experienced ❑ Need practice ❑ Never done ❑ Not applicable (based on scope of practice)	❑ Verbal ❑ Demonstration/ observation ❑ Practical exercise ❑ Interactive class	❑ Beginner ❑ Intermediate ❑ Expert	❑ Orientation ❑ Annual ❑ Other _____	

Employee signature

Observer signature

Reference:

Perry, A. and Potter, P. 2006. *Clinical Nursing Skills & Techniques.* 6th Ed. St. Louis, MO: Mosby.

Name: ______________________ Date: ______________

Skill: **Blood Glucose Meter**

Steps	Completed	Comments
1. Demonstrates how to properly clean meter.		
2. Turns on meter and correctly verifies test strip code.		
3. Performs check strip validation correctly.		
4. Performs high & low controls according to instructions/prompts.		
5. Explains or demonstrates how to appropriately document quality control (QC) results (QC log).		
6. Explains or demonstrates how to correct a "failed" QC result.		
7. Explains/demonstrates how to document the corrective action on a "failed" QC result.		
Patient testing		
1. Properly identifies patient.		
2. Describes procedure to patient.		
3. Wears appropriate personal protective equipment (PPE) when collecting/handling sample.		
4. Assesses patient's fingertips and chooses appropriate site for sample collection.		
5. Explains or demonstrates purpose of test code chip and how to replace.		
6. Turns on meter and verifies test strip code correctly.		
7. Correctly inserts test strip into meter.		
8. Correctly obtains blood sample from fingerstick.		
9. Applies sufficient amount of blood sample to test strip.		
10. Documents patient result on appropriate form/chart.		
11. Provides appropriate postfingerstick care to patient.		
12. Discards testing materials in appropriate containers (i.e., lancet, test strip, etc.).		

13. States critical value ranges when a sample is to be collected and sent to the laboratory for analysis.		
14. Explains or demonstrates the collection of a confirmation sample.		
15. Reviewed current procedure for relevant revisions.		

Self-assessment	Evaluation/ validation methods	Levels	Type of validation	Comments
❑ Experienced ❑ Need practice ❑ Never done ❑ Not applicable (based on scope of practice)	❑ Verbal ❑ Demonstration/ observation ❑ Practical exercise ❑ Interactive class	❑ Beginner ❑ Intermediate ❑ Expert	❑ Orientation ❑ Annual ❑ Other _____	

______________________________ ______________________________

Employee signature ***Observer signature***

Reference:

Duell, D., Martin, B., and Smith, S. 2008. *Clinical Nursing Skills: Basic to Advanced Skills*. 7th ed. Upper Saddle River, NJ: Pearson Education, Inc.

Name: ______________________________ Date: ______________

Skill: **Blood Pressure Measurement—Automatic**

Steps	Completed	Comments
1. Identifies patient and explains procedure.		
2. Selects an appropriately sized blood-pressure cuff for the patient, attaches to machine.		
3. Locates the brachial artery (inner aspect of the elbow) and feels for pulse.		
4. Places cuff so the inflatable bag is centered over the brachial artery and the lower edge of the cuff is 1-2 inches above pulse site.		
5. Wraps cuff around the arm snugly; fastens it securely.		
6. Places patient's arm in position of comfort, relaxed at or below level of patient's heart.		
7. Turns Monitor "ON," and pushes Start button.		
8. Reads Blood Pressure accurately and reports to patient's nurse if outside expected measurement for patient, or normal range.		
9. Records measurement in PLATO or on paper graphic if PLATO is not available.		
10. Removes cuff, and places patient in position of comfort and safety.		

Self-assessment	Evaluation/ validation methods	Levels	Type of validation	Comments
❑ Experienced ❑ Need practice ❑ Never done ❑ Not applicable (based on scope of practice)	❑ Verbal ❑ Demonstration/ observation ❑ Practical exercise ❑ Interactive class	❑ Beginner ❑ Intermediate ❑ Expert	❑ Orientation ❑ Annual ❑ Other _____	

_________________________ _________________________

Employee signature *Observer signature*

Reference:

Duell, D., Martin, B., and Smith, S. 2008. *Clinical Nursing Skills: Basic to Advanced Skills*. 7th ed. Upper Saddle River, NJ: Pearson Education, Inc.

Name: ______________________________ Date: ______________

Skill: **Blood Pressure Measurement—Manual**

Steps	Completed	Comments
1. Identifies patient and explains procedure.		
2. Selects an appropriately sized blood-pressure cuff for the patient.		
3. Locates the brachial artery (inner aspect of the elbow).		
4. Places cuff so the inflatable bag is centered over the brachial artery and the lower edge of the cuff is about one to two inches above site.		
5. Wraps cuff around the arm snugly; fastens it securely or tucks the end of the cuff well under the preceding wrapping.		
6. Places the stethoscope into ears and closes the screw valve on the air pump.		
7. With the fingertips of left hand, feels for the pulse over brachial artery. Places stethoscope firmly but with little pressure over area.		
8. Palpates brachial artery with left hand and pumps bulb until gauge rises about 30 mmHg above the point at which the brachial pulse disappears, or pumps bulb until gauge is 30 mmHg above the point that the BP has been running.		
9. Uses the valve on the bulb to release air slowly, and notes the point on the manometer at which the first of two consecutive beats is heard (systolic pressure).		
10. Continues to release air in the cuff evenly and slowly. Notes the reading on the manometer when all sounds disappear (diastolic pressure).		
11. Allows the remaining air to escape quickly and removes the cuff.		
12. Documents blood pressure reading on graphic record.		

Self-assessment	Evaluation/ validation methods	Levels	Type of validation	Comments
❑ Experienced ❑ Need practice ❑ Never done ❑ Not applicable (based on scope of practice)	❑ Verbal ❑ Demonstration/ observation ❑ Practical exercise ❑ Interactive class	❑ Beginner ❑ Intermediate ❑ Expert	❑ Orientation ❑ Annual ❑ Other _____	

_______________________________ *Employee signature*

_______________________________ *Observer signature*

Reference:

Duell, D., Martin, B., and Smith, S. 2008. ***Clinical Nursing Skills: Basic to Advanced Skills***. 7th ed. Upper Saddle River, NJ: Pearson Education, Inc.

Name: ______________________________ Date: ______________

Skill: **Diagnostic Cardiology—Digital Holter Hook-up**

Steps	Completed	Comments
UPLOADING STUDIES		
1. Demonstrate verification of patient recording (serial number or diary return).		
2. Demonstrate use of Load screen…logging appropriate information.		
3. Demonstrate physical connection to computer.		
4. Demonstrate send to out-box function.		
5. Demonstrate removal of battery.		
6. Demonstrate proper cleaning of recorder and cable.		
DOWNLOADING REPORTS		
1. Demonstrate understanding and navigation between in-box and archive.		
2. Demonstrate retrieval from in-box to view.		
3. Demonstrate view and print reverse order functions.		
4. Demonstrate move from in-box to archive function.		
5. Demonstrate reconciliation between charts and reports.		
6. Demonstrate reconciliation between reports and recorders.		

Self-assessment	Evaluation/ validation methods	Levels	Type of validation	Comments
❑ Experienced ❑ Need practice ❑ Never done ❑ Not applicable (based on scope of practice)	❑ Verbal ❑ Demonstration/ observation ❑ Practical exercise ❑ Interactive class	❑ Beginner ❑ Intermediate ❑ Expert	❑ Orientation ❑ Annual ❑ Other _____	

______________________________ ______________________________

Employee signature ***Observer signature***

Reference:

Nissen, S., Pepine, C., Bashore, T., et al. 1994. American College of Cardiology position statement. Cardiac angiography without cine film: erecting a "tower of Babel" in the cardiac catheterization laboratory. *Journal of the American College of Cardiology* 24: 834-837.

Name: ______________________________ Date: ______________

Skill: **Emergency Preparedness**

Steps	Completed	Comments
1. Assesses if a medical emergency exists: physical assessment (patient responsiveness, LOC, vitals); historical assessment (diabetes, autonomic neuropathy, hypotensive episodes).		
2. Identifies correct pathway cardiac rehab emergency treatment algorithm.		
3. Demonstrates ventilation technique via Resusci mask.		
4. Demonstrates O^2 to ambu bag and nasal cannula hook-up.		
5. Demonstrates fitting patient with nasal cannula.		
6. Performs BLS ABCs and one cycle of rescue breathing and cardiac compressions.		
7. Identifies team code number to call.		
8. Demonstrates technique for transferring patient from telemetry to defibrillator leads, selects limb and augmented lead positions, runs an ECG strip.		
9. Transports team cart and gurney from exam room to exercise area.		
10. Identifies team cart components: emergency drug box, phase IV solutions, IV start sets, pulse oximeter.		
11. Demonstrates: placement of conductive defib pads on the chest wall, placement and pressure on the defib paddles, and the correct sequence of ACLS defibrillation shocks.		
12. Demonstrates technique for transferring patient to gurney and transporting patient to exam room or ED.		

Self-assessment	Evaluation/ validation methods	Levels	Type of validation	Comments
❑ Experienced ❑ Need practice ❑ Never done ❑ Not applicable (based on scope of practice)	❑ Verbal ❑ Demonstration/ observation ❑ Practical exercise ❑ Interactive class	❑ Beginner ❑ Intermediate ❑ Expert	❑ Orientation ❑ Annual ❑ Other _____	

Employee signature ***Observer signature***

Reference:

Gazmuri, R. et al. 2007. Scientific knowledge gaps and clinical research priorities for cardiopulmonary resuscitation and emergency cardiac care identified during the 2005 international consensus conference on E and CPR science with treatment recommendations: A consensus statement from the International Liaison Committee on Resuscitation, the American Heart Association Emergency Cardiovascular Care Committee, the Stroke Council and Cardiovascular Nursing Council. *Circulation* 116: 2501-2512.

Name: ______________________________ Date: ______________

Skill: **Falls Prevention—Get Up and Go**

Steps	Completed	Comments
1. Verbalize three factors related to hospitalization which increase the risk of falls for elderly in the hospital.		
2. Demonstrate the steps of the Get Up and Go Test, as if the patient. a. Have the patient sit in a chair b. Instruct the patient to stand up c. Ask the patient to stand still with eyes open d. Ask patient to close eyes and stand still e. Instruct patient to open eyes and walk 10 feet, turn around and come back f. Ask patient to sit down in the chair again		
3. Verbalize at least one factor to assess during each step of the testing.		
4. Differentiate the timed results of the test as to risk for falls. Be able to state: a. Less than 20 seconds is low risk b. 20-30 seconds moderate risk c. Greater than 30 seconds is high risk		
5. List at least 5 nursing interventions for falls prevention.		

Self-assessment	Evaluation/ validation methods	Levels	Type of validation	Comments
❑ Experienced ❑ Need practice ❑ Never done ❑ Not applicable (based on scope of practice)	❑ Verbal ❑ Demonstration/ observation ❑ Practical exercise ❑ Interactive class	❑ Beginner ❑ Intermediate ❑ Expert	❑ Orientation ❑ Annual ❑ Other _____	

______________________________ ______________________________

Employee signature *Observer signature*

Reference:

American Geriatrics Society, British Geriatrics Society, and American Academy of Orthopaedic Surgeons Panel on Falls Prevention. 2001. Guidelines for the prevention of falls in older persons. *Journal of the American Geriatrics Society* 49(5): 664-672.

Name: ____________________ Date: ____________

Skill: **Fit Testing for N-95 Respirator Masks**

Steps	Completed	Comments
1. Identifies if the employee has completed the Respiratory Questionnaire. Notes what (if any) answers on the questionnaire would indicate the employee should not be Fit Tested. (Based on the OSHA Respiratory Protection Standards.)		
2. Explains the Fit Test Procedure to the employee.		
3. Performs the Fit test per the OSHA Respiratory Protection Standards. Performs a Sensitivity Check on the employee with either saccharin solution or bitrex solution. Appropriately uses bitrex solution if the employee cannot taste the saccharin solution. Assists the employee to put on the N-95 respirator mask, coaching the employee on assuring a good tight fit and how to adjust the mask as appropriate. Performs the Fit Test on the employee (noting each step that should be carried out during the testing process – regular breathing, deep breathing, turning head from side to side, nodding up and down, talking, grimacing and frowning, and smiling). Assists the employee to readjust their mask if needed during the process. Verbalizes when another mask should be used in the Fit Test procedure. Explains to the employee when to wear their mask.		

Self-assessment	Evaluation/ validation methods	Levels	Type of validation	Comments
❑ Experienced ❑ Need practice ❑ Never done ❑ Not applicable (based on scope of practice)	❑ Verbal ❑ Demonstration/ observation ❑ Practical exercise ❑ Interactive class	❑ Beginner ❑ Intermediate ❑ Expert	❑ Orientation ❑ Annual ❑ Other _____	

Employee signature

Observer signature

Reference:

United States Department of Labor Occupational Safety and Health Administration. Fit testing guidelines. Standards 29CFR 1910.134, Appendix A.

Name: ______________________________ Date: ________________

Skill: **Intake and Output**

Steps	Completed	Comments
1. Diet: Estimates % of diet eaten from tray each meal. Records amount of taken in on door as tray is removed from room.		
2. Fluids: Identifies number of cc's taken in by patient in the form of liquids, pop, jello, or ice. Locates and uses unit reference for fluids as necessary. Documents on door slip for appropriate shift.		
3. Output: Using proper PPE empties and measures amount of urine in bedpan or urinal, or foley.		
4. Disposes of urine. Washes hands.		
5. Record amount of urine on door slip.		

Self-assessment	Evaluation/ validation methods	Levels	Type of validation	Comments
❑ Experienced ❑ Need practice ❑ Never done ❑ Not applicable (based on scope of practice)	❑ Verbal ❑ Demonstration/ observation ❑ Practical exercise ❑ Interactive class	❑ Beginner ❑ Intermediate ❑ Expert	❑ Orientation ❑ Annual ❑ Other _____	

_______________________________ _______________________________

Employee signature *Observer signature*

Reference:

Alvare, S., Dugan, D., and Fuzy, J. 2005. *Nursing Assistant Care*. Albuquerque, NM: Hartman Publishing.

Name: ______________________ Date: ______________

Skill: **Medication Administration**

Steps	Completed	Comments
Routine Medications:		
1. Verifies all pages of the MAR/Medication Record are present. a. When giving the first dose of any medication checks for last dose given of a similar-acting medication so appropriate time interval can be maintained.		
2. Takes MAR & COW to verify and prepare medications.		
3. Identify the patient by checking the following: a. Patient name and medical record number/birthday on identification band with patient name and medical record number on MAR.		
4. **Check allergies each time a medication is administered. Identify allergies by checking:** **a. For red allergy arm band** **b. For documentation of allergies on MAR, Home Medication List, FACT Sheet, or on History & Physical. Electronic chart utilize information tab or header.**		
5. Check the label sent with pharmacy against MAR; if it does not match, a check of the order is done.		
6. Check when giving the first dose of any medication for last dose given of a similar-acting medication so appropriate time interval can be maintained.		
7. Opens unit-dose packaging at the bedside when patient is ready to take the medication. Places medication in a cup or directly in the patient's hand. a. Takes pill cutter or crusher to bedside **and splits or crushes medication at the bedside**. b. Uses appropriate syringe if patient has Dobhoff/NGT.		

8. **Stays with the patient until medication is administered and does not leave medication at bedside unless ordered.**		
9. When administering oral medications, raises the patient to a sitting position if condition permits. Gives sufficient fluid to facilitate swallowing.		
10. Sanitize hands.		
11. Documents **after** medication is given with initial.		
12. If the medication is NOT given, circles time and initials. **Indicates the reason for omission on MAR/medication record.** a. **If medication is given late, documents time med was given.**		
13. **Signs each sheet of the MAR or medication record in appropriate shift block.**		
14. **Documents fluid intake amount (IV or PO) if patient on I & O record.**		

Self-assessment	Evaluation/ validation methods	Levels	Type of validation	Comments
❑ Experienced ❑ Need practice ❑ Never done ❑ Not applicable (based on scope of practice)	❑ Verbal ❑ Demonstration/ observation ❑ Practical exercise ❑ Interactive class	❑ Beginner ❑ Intermediate ❑ Expert	❑ Orientation ❑ Annual ❑ Other _____	

_______________________________ _______________________________

Employee signature *Observer signature*

Reference:

Perry, A. and Potter, P. 2006. *Clinical Nursing Skills & Techniques*. 6th Ed. St. Louis, MO: Mosby Elsevier.

Name: ____________________ Date: ____________

Skill: **Oxygen Administration**

Steps	Completed	Comments
1. Verifies the physician's order.		
2. Washes hands.		
3. Obtains the required equipment: a. Oxygen flowmeter b. Humidifier (over 4 liters) c. Sterile water (over 4 liters) d. Oxygen connecting tubing (if needed) e. Oxygen administration device		
4. Identifies the patient and explains procedure.		
5. Adjusts the device to the ordered level.		
6. Applies the device to the patient.		
7. Confirms FiO2 as appropriate.		
8. Leaves the patient area clean and safe after disposing of excess equipment.		
9. Washes hands before leaving room.		
10. Documents equipment, concentration, or liter flow in the patient's chart.		

Self-assessment	Evaluation/ validation methods	Levels	Type of validation	Comments
❑ Experienced ❑ Need practice ❑ Never done ❑ Not applicable (based on scope of practice)	❑ Verbal ❑ Demonstration/ observation ❑ Practical exercise ❑ Interactive class	❑ Beginner ❑ Intermediate ❑ Expert	❑ Orientation ❑ Annual ❑ Other _____	

________________________ ________________________

Employee signature *Observer signature*

Reference:

Duell, D., Martin, B., and Smith, S. 2008. *Clinical Nursing Skills: Basic to Advanced Skills.* 7th ed. New Jersey: Pearson Education, Inc.

Perry, A. and Potter, P. 2006. *Clinical Nursing Skills & Techniques.* 6th Ed. St. Louis, MO: Mosby Elsevier.

Name: ______________________________ Date: ______________

Skill: **Presentation Skills**

Steps	Completed	Comments
1. Uses appropriate teaching methods for content being taught.		
2. Speaks clearly.		
3. Presents in organized manner.		
4. Maintains eye contact.		
5. Presents at the level of the learner.		
6. Summarizes material.		
7. Encourages audience participation.		
8. Correlates theory to practice.		
9. Generates learner questions.		
10. Gives participants opportunity to evaluate program.		
11. Administers and reviews pre- and posttests with the participants.		

Self-assessment	Evaluation/ validation methods	Levels	Type of validation	Comments
❑ Experienced ❑ Need practice ❑ Never done ❑ Not applicable (based on scope of practice)	❑ Verbal ❑ Demonstration/ observation ❑ Practical exercise ❑ Interactive class	❑ Beginner ❑ Intermediate ❑ Expert	❑ Orientation ❑ Annual ❑ Other _____	

______________________________ ______________________________

Employee signature ***Observer signature***

Reference:

Brunt, B. 2007. *Competencies for Staff Educators: Tools to Evaluate and Enhance Nursing Professional Development*. Marblehead, MA: HCPro, Inc.

Name: ______________________________ Date: ______________

Skill: **Regulating and Maintaining Proper IV Rate**

Steps	Completed	Comments
Observations to be made during IV infusion. A. Initial shift assessment identifies: 1. Correct fluid is handling. 2. Infusing at correct rate. 3. Verifies all pump settings are correct. 4. All connections are intact. 5. IV tubing off floor. 6. No kinks in tubing. 7. Drip chamber with correct fluid level. 8. Dressing occlusive. 9. IV site clear, without redness or swelling (benign). 10. Dates on tubing/dressing of initiation. 11. Verbalized date of site, tubing and dressing changes.		
B. Assessment to be made q1° 1. IV running at correct rate. 2. All pump settings correct. 3. IV site benign. 4. Tubing intact and without kinks.		

Self-assessment	Evaluation/ validation methods	Levels	Type of validation	Comments
❏ Experienced ❏ Need practice ❏ Never done ❏ Not applicable (based on scope of practice)	❏ Verbal ❏ Demonstration/ observation ❏ Practical exercise ❏ Interactive class	❏ Beginner ❏ Intermediate ❏ Expert	❏ Orientation ❏ Annual ❏ Other _____	

______________________________ ______________________________

Employee signature *Observer signature*

Reference:

Weinstein, S. 2007. *Plumer's Principles and Practice of Intravenous Therapy*. 8th ed. Philadelphia, PA: Lippincott.

Name: ______________________________ Date: ______________

Skill: **Service Excellence/Patient Satisfaction**

Steps	Completed	Comments
Uses the "3 Cs" principles of caring, concern, and communication by following AIDET:		
1. Acknowledges patient by name; makes eye contact; asks "is there anything I can do for you?"		
2. Introduces self by name and skillset, professional certification, and experience.		
3. Duration gives an accurate time expectation for tests, tray delivery, and/or physician arrival.		
4. Explains step by step what will happen, answers questions; leaves phone number or method to reach you. Assures privacy. Connects key words with patient safety and excellent care.		
5. Thanks the patient for choosing Summa; expresses concern for inconvenience often caused by healthcare experience. Thanks the patient's family for assistance and support of the patient.		

Self-assessment	Evaluation/ validation methods	Levels	Type of validation	Comments
❑ Experienced ❑ Need practice ❑ Never done ❑ Not applicable (based on scope of practice)	❑ Verbal ❑ Demonstration/ observation ❑ Practical exercise ❑ Interactive class	❑ Beginner ❑ Intermediate ❑ Expert	❑ Orientation ❑ Annual ❑ Other _____	

______________________________ ______________________________

Employee signature ***Observer signature***

Reference:

Studer, Q. 2003. *Hardwiring Excellence.* Gulf Breeze, FL: Fire Starter Publishing.

Name: ______________________ Date: ______________

Skill: **Thrombolytic Therapy**

Steps	Completed	Comments
Before therapy is begun: 1. Established 2 vascular access sites (one may be HL) and checks sites at least q 15 min.		
2. Verbalized contraindications. (Uncontrolled hypertension, history of bleeding ulcer, active internal bleeding, recent intracranial/intraspinal surgery or trauma, intracranial neoplasm, AV malformation, aneurysm.)		
3. Uses caution/gentleness when moving patient.		
4. Obtains baseline VS and neuron status.		
5. Obtains baseline laboratory values (Hemogram, PT, PTT, fibrinogen, electrolytes, CPK).		
6. Avoids repeated needle punctures (blood draws are grouped, avoid IM injections if possible).		
During therapy infusion: 1. Monitor VS and neuron status q 15 min and notifies physician of change immediately.		
2. Checks arm under blood pressure cuff for ecchymosis q 1 hour. Rotates cuff prn.		
3. Monitor for signs of reperfusion (decreased chest pain, resolution of ST elevation, development of arrhythmias).		
4. Looks for subtle signs of bleeding (tachycardia, orthostatic hypotension).		
5. Assess all body drainage for presence of blood findings (urine/stool/emesis/gastric drainage).		
6. Monitors lab values (H&H, PT, PTT, other coag, BUN, Creat, Cardiac markers).		
7. Applies pressure to all venipuncture sites for at least 5 minutes.		
8. Identifies risk factors for clot information (elderly, diabetic, smoking hs., elevated lipids, hypertension, sedentary lifestyle).		
After therapy is completed: 1. Monitors VS and neuron check's q 15 min x 2 hr then q 1 hr x 2 then q 2 hr. x 24hrs.		

2. Monitors lab values using 2nd IV site q 12 hr x 24 hr then qd x2.		
3. Assess for subtle signs of bleeding (as above) q 12 hr.		
4. Assess for signs of reocclusion and notifies physician immediately (Recurrent chest pain, ST segment elevation, diaphoresis, nausea, arrhythmia).		
5. Educates the patient about the current therapy and also the probable use of a "blood thinner" at home (Coumadin booklet).		

Self-assessment	Evaluation/ validation methods	Levels	Type of validation	Comments
❑ Experienced ❑ Need practice ❑ Never done ❑ Not applicable (based on scope of practice)	❑ Verbal ❑ Demonstration/ observation ❑ Practical exercise ❑ Interactive class	❑ Beginner ❑ Intermediate ❑ Expert	❑ Orientation ❑ Annual ❑ Other _____	

Employee signature ***Observer signature***

Reference:

American College of Cardiology and the American Heart Association. *ACC/AHA Guideline for the Management of Patients With ST-Elevation Myocardial Infarction Pocket Guide.* 2004.

Name: ______________________________ Date: ______________

Skill: **Thrombus: Chronic versus Acute**

Steps	Completed	Comments
1. Performs venous duplex study according to protocol.		
2. Reviews patient chart for previous DVT, PE history.		
3. Observes and documents for acute DVT: • Dilatation of vessel • Sonolucent echoes with difficulty compressing • No or poor spontaneous flow • Poor augmention		
4. Observes and documents for chronic DVT: • Recanalization • Heterogeneous or bright echoes • Collaterals • Small vessel or atrophy of vessel • Incompetency of valves • Patient history of previous DVT, PE		

Self-assessment	Evaluation/ validation methods	Levels	Type of validation	Comments
❑ Experienced ❑ Need practice ❑ Never done ❑ Not applicable (based on scope of practice)	❑ Verbal ❑ Demonstration/ observation ❑ Practical exercise ❑ Interactive class	❑ Beginner ❑ Intermediate ❑ Expert	❑ Orientation ❑ Annual ❑ Other _____	

______________________________ ______________________________

Employee signature *Observer signature*

Reference:

National Heart Lung and Blood Institute. 2007. *Deep vein thrombosis.* United States Department of Health and Human Services.

Name: ______________________________ Date: ______________

Skill: **Use of Automated External Defibrillator (Heartstream FR2)**

Steps	Completed	Comments
1. Assesses the patient for unconsciousness, no breathing, and no detectable pulse.		
2. Turns on the Heartstream FR2.		
3. Simulates proper skin prep prior to pads placement.		
4. Correctly places defibrillation pads.		
5. Plugs the pads connector into Heartstream FR2's connector port.		
6. Ensures no one touches the patient when Heartstream FR2 is analyzing.		
7. Verbally and visually clears the patient prior to delivering shock.		
8. Presses shock button when advised.		
9. Assesses patient for presence of a pulse when the Heartstream FR2 gives a "No Shock Advised" message.		

Self-assessment	Evaluation/ validation methods	Levels	Type of validation	Comments
❑ Experienced ❑ Need practice ❑ Never done ❑ Not applicable (based on scope of practice)	❑ Verbal ❑ Demonstration/ observation ❑ Practical exercise ❑ Interactive class	❑ Beginner ❑ Intermediate ❑ Expert	❑ Orientation ❑ Annual ❑ Other _____	

_______________________________ _______________________________

Employee signature *Observer signature*

Reference:

American Heart Association. 2005. American Heart Association guidelines for cardiopulmonary resuscitation and emergency cardiovascular care. *Circulation* 112: IV35-IV46.

Name: ______________________________ Date: ______________

Skill: **Venipuncture with Winged Needle**

Steps	Completed	Comments
1. Washes hands.		
2. Obtains IV tray ensuring equipment is present (winged needle, prep swabs, tourniquet, dressing, and tape).		
3. Organizes and prepares: a. Winged needle b. Prep swabs (alcohol or bedadine) c. Tourniquet d. Tape e. Dressing f. Towel or disposable blue underpad g. Gloves		
4. Explains procedure to patient.		
5. Identifies site, stating criteria for selection (avoids bony prominences, wrist, and dominate hand and uses most distal vein).		
6. Dons gloves.		
7. Selects size winged needle and states criteria for selection.		
8. Places tourniquet 5–6″ above site to obstruct venous flow only.		
9. Selects vein.		
10. Cleanses site (from center out using betadine or alcohol).		
11. Removes cap from needle.		
12. Holds hand or forearm with nondominant hand and secures vein beneath insertion site with thumb.		
13. Places needle bevel up at 30–45 ° angle from skin and punctures vein.		
14. Observes blood return.		
15. Advances winged needle into vein an additional one-quarter to one-half inch		
16. Releases tourniquet.		
17. Attaches IV tubing.		

18. Applies IV dressing.		
19. Tapes IV tubing.		
20. Labels IV dressing.		
21. Labels IV tubing.		
22. Removes gloves and discards.		
23. Washes hands.		
24. States appropriate number of times allowed for venipuncture, if unsuccessful, and steps to take once that number has been reached.		
25. Documents procedure.		

Self-assessment	Evaluation/ validation methods	Levels	Type of validation	Comments
❑ Experienced ❑ Need practice ❑ Never done ❑ Not applicable (based on scope of practice)	❑ Verbal ❑ Demonstration/ observation ❑ Practical exercise ❑ Interactive class	❑ Beginner ❑ Intermediate ❑ Expert	❑ Orientation ❑ Annual ❑ Other _____	

_______________________________ _______________________________

Employee signature ***Observer signature***

Reference:

Weinstein, S. 2007. *Plumer's Principles and Practice of Intravenous Therapy*. 8th ed. Philadelphia, PA: Lippincott.

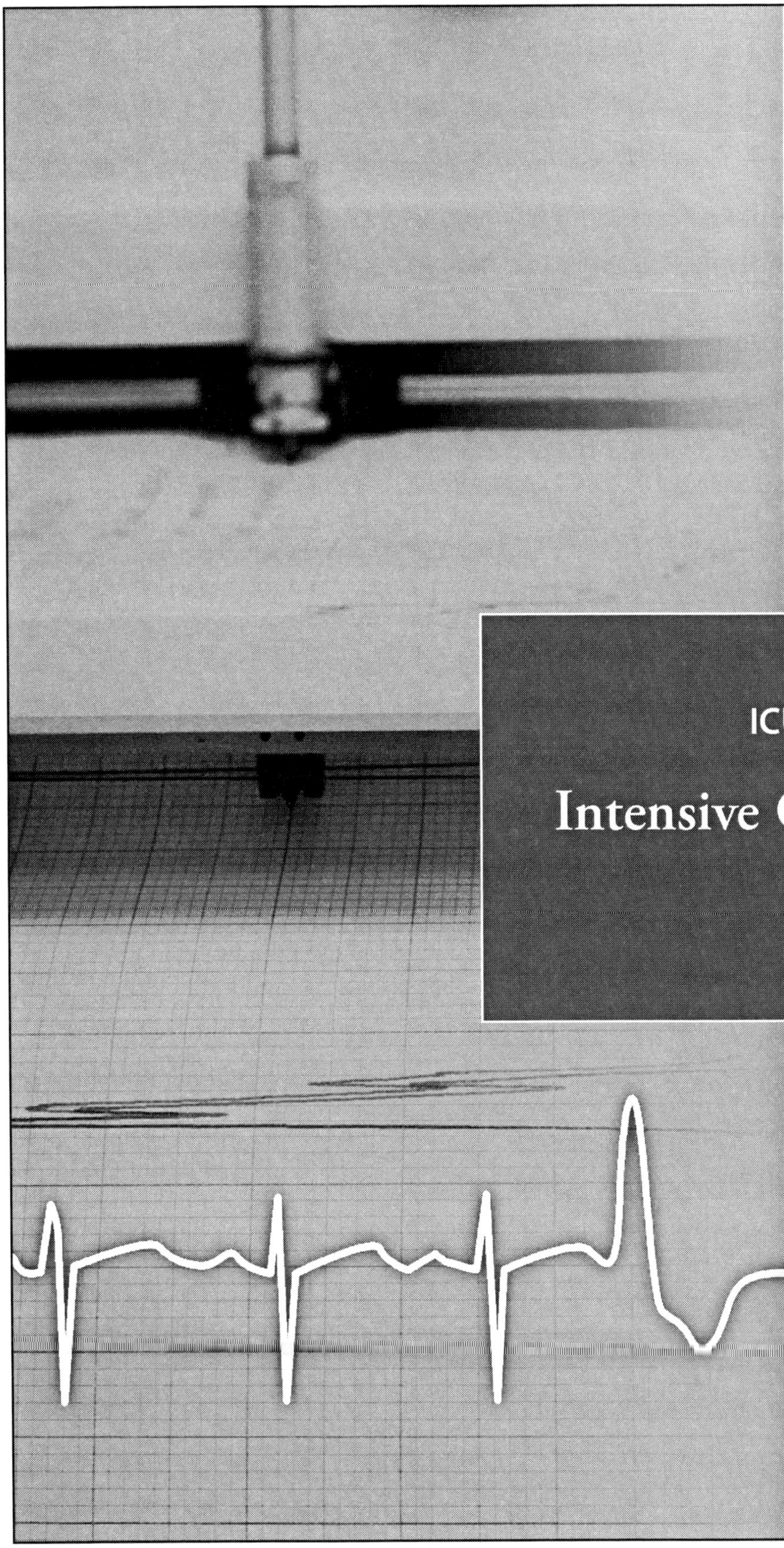

ICU

Intensive Care Unit

Contents

Name: ______________________________ Date: ______________

Skill: **Arterial Duplex Graft**

Steps	Completed	Comments
1. Check the physician order. Obtain the operative report to note the location of the proximal and distal graft anastomosis. Document the patient history including risk factors of ASO and previous surgery.		
2. Scan the entire length of the graft in transverse view noting abnormalities such as: stenosis, perigraft fluid, aneurismal dilatation, intraluminal defect, or tributaries (insitu grafts). Use color flow to assist.		
3. Scan in longitudinal view with color starting in the native artery, proximal to the proximal anastomosis. Follow the entire graft to the distal anastomosis and into the outflow artery.		
4. Obtain peak systolic velocities in the long view using a 60 degree angle or less at: the inflow artery, proximal anastomosis, upper thigh, mid thigh, distal thigh, knee area, upper calf, mid-distal calf, distal anastomosis and outflow artery. Also evaluate velocities at any area of color aliasing or areas of stenosis.		
5. Obtain bilateral ankle PVR waveforms. Obtain bilateral brachial and ankle BP and perform an ankle/brachial index.		
6. Document on the worksheet the date, patient demographics, videotape number, graft location, PVR waveforms, ABI's and technician comments.		

Self-assessment	Evaluation/ validation methods	Levels	Type of validation	Comments
❑ Experienced ❑ Need practice ❑ Never done ❑ Not applicable (based on scope of practice)	❑ Verbal ❑ Demonstration/ observation ❑ Practical exercise ❑ Interactive class	❑ Beginner ❑ Intermediate ❑ Expert	❑ Orientation ❑ Annual ❑ Other _____	

_______________________ _______________________

Employee signature *Observer signature*

Reference:
Calabrese, D. and Modic, M. "Renal and Urologic Care" in *Nursing Procedures*. 3rd ed. Springhouse, PA: Springhouse Corporation. 595-597.

Name: ______________________________ Date: ______________

Skill: **Arterial Line Monitoring**

Steps	Completed	Comments
A. Arterial line set-up.		
1. Uses principles of BSI.		
2. Assembles arterial line equipment: a. Labels flush bag and tubing with date, time, and initials. b. Connects pressure tubing to NS flush bag. c. Flushes tubing/stopcocks to remove all air from system. d. Replaces vented white caps with blue dead-ender caps e. Sets pressure infusor at 300 mmHg.		
B. Obtaining blood specimens from an arterial line.		
ACH a. Removes dead-ender, attaches vacutainer adapter with holder to stopcock. (May replace blue dead-ender with leur lock,) b. Turns stopcock off to transducer, fills medium red top tube and discards. c. Attaches and fills appropriate tubes. d. Turns stopcock off to the open port, flushes catheter. e. Turns stopcock off to patient and detaches vacutainer adapter with holder; flushes port, or leur lock; turns stopcock off to the open port and places sterile dead-ender or leur lock. Rezeros transducer.		
STH a. Fills VAMP chamber. b. Turns stopcock off to the chamber. c. Attaches vacutainer adapter with holder to port. d. Attaches and fills appropriate tubes. e. Removes vacutainer with holder. f. Turns stopcock open to the patient and replaces aspirated blood/flush catheter.		
C. Removal of an arterial line catheter		
1. Uses principles of BSI.		

2. Turns alarms off. Disconnects transducer from monitor.		
3. Opens 4x4, sterile suture set.		
4. Removes dressing, assesses site, removes sutures.		
5. Withdraws catheter while maintaining pressure over site.		
6. Immediately applies firm pressure for a minimum of five minutes and until bleeding stops. • Radial • Femoral		
7. Applies povidone iodine ointment and pressure dressing to site.		
8. Describes care of arterial site s/p line removal. • Radial. • Femoral.		
D. Maintenance and monitoring of an arterial line catheter.		
1. Checks arterial line pressure with cuff pressure q shift.		
2. Observes and documents arterial wave form for patency, position, and blood pressure reading q1°hr.		
3. Checks neuro vascular status of extremity distal arterial line insertion site q1°hr.		
4. Changes tubing/pressurized solution bag and dressing q72 hr. (LPN's may not change tubing once attached to patient; may perform dressing change.)		

Self-assessment	Evaluation/ validation methods	Levels	Type of validation	Comments
❑ Experienced ❑ Need practice ❑ Never done ❑ Not applicable (based on scope of practice)	❑ Verbal ❑ Demonstration/ observation ❑ Practical exercise ❑ Interactive class	❑ Beginner ❑ Intermediate ❑ Expert	❑ Orientation ❑ Annual ❑ Other _____	

_______________________________ _______________________________

Employee signature ***Observer signature***

Reference:

Carlson, K. and Weigand, D. 2005. *AACN Procedure Manual for Critical Care*. 5th ed. St. Louis, MO: Elsevier Saunders.

Name: ____________________ Date: ____________

Skill: **Barthel Index Modified Rankin Scale**

Steps	Completed	Comments
1. Selects the appropriate score for the patient using the Barthel Index Scoring System (5, 10, 15) for each area of activity:		
A. Feeding		
B. Bathing		
C. Grooming		
D. Dressing		
E. Bowel control		
F. Bladder control		
G. Toilet transfers		
H. Chair/bed transfers		
I. Ambulation		
J. Stairs		
2. Records performance in each category prior to admission and on admission by interviewing patient or family, if not already obtained.		
3. Enters total Barthel Index Score and initials.		
4. Enters Modified Rankin Scale score as indicated by patient's physical limitations into appropriate box.		
5. Enters initials as appropriate.		

Self-assessment	Evaluation/ validation methods	Levels	Type of validation	Comments
❑ Experienced ❑ Need practice ❑ Never done ❑ Not applicable (based on scope of practice)	❑ Verbal ❑ Demonstration/ observation ❑ Practical exercise ❑ Interactive class	❑ Beginner ❑ Intermediate ❑ Expert	❑ Orientation ❑ Annual ❑ Other _____	

Employee signature ____________________

Observer signature ____________________

Reference:

Barthel, D., and Mahoney, F. 1965. Functional evaluation: the Barthel Index. *Maryland State Medical Journal* 14: 56-61.

Name: ______________________ Date: ______________

Skill: **Bipolar ECG Identification—Cardiac Rehab**

Steps	Completed	Comments
1. Identifies the normal time components and configuration of a. P Wave b. QRS complex c. ST segment d. T wave		
2. Identifies/describes the key ECG components of a. Normal sinus rhythm b. Sinus bradycardia c. Sinus tachycardia.		
3. Identifies/describes the components of the following abnormal ECGs: a. Premature atrial complex b. Premature ventricular complex c. Premature junctional complex d. Ventricular tachycardia e. Supraventricular tachycardia f. Ventricular fibrillation g. Atrial fibrillation h. Atrial flutter		
4. Identifies/describes a misplaced or transposed ECG electrode configuration.		
5. Identifies/illustrates the following ECG conduction defects: a. Bundle branch block b. First degree av block c. Second degree av block (mobitz i) d. Second degree av block (mobitz ii) e. Third degree av block		

Self-assessment	Evaluation/ validation methods	Levels	Type of validation	Comments
❑ Experienced ❑ Need practice ❑ Never done ❑ Not applicable (based on scope of practice)	❑ Verbal ❑ Demonstration/ observation ❑ Practical exercise ❑ Interactive class	❑ Beginner ❑ Intermediate ❑ Expert	❑ Orientation ❑ Annual ❑ Other _____	

_______________________ _______________________

Employee signature *Observer signature*

Reference:

American Heart Association. 2005. Guidelines for cardiopulmonary resuscitation and emergency cardiovascular care. *Circulation* 112(Supp. 24): IV1-IV211.

Name: ______________________________ Date: ______________

Skill: **Camino Intracranial Pressure Monitoring**

Steps	Completed	Comments
I. Insertion and set-up		
1. Assembles appropriate equipment.		
2. Labels bedside monitor to calculate CPP.		
3. Labels monitor for ICP.		
4. Zeroes and calibrates bedside monitor and Camino monitor.		
5. Maintains aseptic technique with all core associated Z device.		
6. Assists physician with bolt insertion.		
7. Secures preamp connector to transducer with tape.		
8. Adjusts transducer connector with adjustment tool to zero transducer.		
9. Assists physician with catheter insertion and verfies ICP waveform on monitor.		
10. Zeroes bedside and Camino monitor after insertion (without adjustment tool).		
II. Nursing care		
1. Maintains sterile technique with dressing change.		
2. Cleanses site with providone-iodine swabs.		
3. Applies betadine ointment to site.		
4. Places precut 2x2 gauze pad around catheter.		
5. Wraps 4x4 pad around catheter and occlusively tapes dressing.		
6. Anchors and secures catheter.		
III. Monitoring		
1. Maintains transducer at level of Foramen of Monroe.		
2. Places ICP precaution sign at bedside.		
3. Recognizes appropriate ICP waveform.		
4. Zeroes and calibrates bedside monitor and Camino monitor QS.		
5. Documents ICP and CPP q 1 hr or as indicated.		

6. Recognizes normal ICP and CPP values.		
7. Recognizes that ICP and CPP trends are more significant than an isolated elevated reading.		

Self-assessment	Evaluation/ validation methods	Levels	Type of validation	Comments
❑ Experienced ❑ Need practice ❑ Never done ❑ Not applicable (based on scope of practice)	❑ Verbal ❑ Demonstration/ observation ❑ Practical exercise ❑ Interactive class	❑ Beginner ❑ Intermediate ❑ Expert	❑ Orientation ❑ Annual ❑ Other _____	

_______________________________ _______________________________

Employee signature ***Observer signature***

Reference:

Fields, L., Blackshear, C., et al. 2005. *Guide to the Patient with Intracranial Pressure Monitoring: AACN Reference Series for Clinical Practice.* Chicago, IL: AACN.

Name: ______________________________ Date: ____________________

Skill: **Code Management—Critical Care**

Steps	Completed	Comments
1. Assesses Responsiveness		
2. If no response calls for help from others on unit. a. If unable to find someone, makes stat call using phone in patient's room. b. Verbalizes correct phone number for Summa's Stat Line.		Ask for cart and AED 757
3. Assesses breathing a. Opens airway		Look, listen and feel > 5 but < 10 sec. Head tilt/ chin lift or jaw thrust.
4. If patient is breathing a. Applies O^2 via NC b. Assess pulse oximetry c. Contacts physician		May (consider) contact Rapid Response Team RN
5. If patient is not breathing provides breaths using bag-valve-mask or barrier device		Check for chest rise
6. Assesses carotid pulse		>5 but <10 seconds
7. If no pulse, begins chest compressions a. Verbalizes compression:ventilation ratio		1 ½ - 2" deep allows for complete chest recoil rate at least 100/min 30:2
8. When cart and second rescuer arrive a. Places backboard under patient b. Turns on AED and follows prompts		Compressions and ventilations continue until AED advises to clear patient
9. Places multifunction pads correctly (or directs placement).		
10. If "no shock advised" per AED, resumes compressions/ventilations.		
11. Assumes role of team leader and assigns rolls and directs care according to current ACLS guidelines. a. Compressor b. Ventilator c. IV d. Defibrillator e. Meds f. Recorder		May turn over leadership role and assume another. Describes possible ways to combine rolls, i.e., IV & Meds.
12. Initiates appropriate drug therapy.		

13. Cardioversion - Considers sedation and analgesic - Turns defibrillator to SYNC - Assures each complex has marker - Charges to appropriate setting - Clears area - Delivers shock - Assesses results - Obtains EKG strip of the event		
14. Transcutaneous Pacing - Sets defibrillator to Pacing mode - Verbalizes rate and output - Assures pacer is sensing - Starts pacing and evaluates capture - Obtains EKG strip of the event - Dials down output until > 100% capture attained at lowest possible output - Assesses patient		Set rate to at least 80 ppm. Output 60mA.
15. After cardiac rhythm and pulse are restored - Assess ABC's & BP - Assure appropriate IV's are running and line remains patent and secure		
16. Assists with endotracheal intubation as needed. - Directs someone to prepare suction - Prepares laryngoscope and lubricates tube - Assures placement - Secures tube - Provides ventilation		No longer than q 6 sec.
17. Participates in postcode debriefing.		
18. Documents entire event on Code Team Record.		
19. Assists with transport of patient to a critical care unit if needed.		

Self-assessment	Evaluation/ validation methods	Levels	Type of validation	Comments
❑ Experienced ❑ Need practice ❑ Never done ❑ Not applicable (based on scope of practice)	❑ Verbal ❑ Demonstration/ observation ❑ Practical exercise ❑ Interactive class	❑ Beginner ❑ Intermediate ❑ Expert	❑ Orientation ❑ Annual ❑ Other _____	

_______________________________ _______________________________

Employee signature ***Observer signature***

Reference:

American Heart Association. 2005. Guidelines for cardiopulmonary resuscitation and emergency cardiovascular care. *Circulation* 112(Supp. 24): IV1-IV211.

Name: ______________________________ Date: ______________

Skill: **Codman External Drainage System II**

Steps	Completed	Comments
General principles 1. Sets up and maintains drainage system.		
2. Monitors dressing and system to assure proper working of system.		
3. Records and verifies amount of drainage q1°.		
4. Maintains and secures drip chamber at desired height as ordered by physician.		
5. Maintains collection bag below level of the patient in a suspended position as opposed to being allowed to lie flat.		
6. Notifies the physician immediately with symptoms of increased intracranial pressure, undue loss of fluid, redness or drainage at skin site.		
7. Posts a sign over the bed to address activity "Before repositioning this patient, please consult nurse staff."		
8. Maintains aseptic technique with all care associated with device.		
Positioning of the drainage bag		
1. Identifies the physician order for the level of the drip chamber.		
2. The zero mark on the chamber must be hung at the ordered level above the insertion site on the patient's head. Uses measuring tape to determine the level.		
3. Secures the system at ordered level.		
4. Makes adjustment of system with changes in patient's position.		
Replacing collection bag 1. Uses side clamps to occlude the tubing proximal to the Luer-lok connection leading to the collection bag.		
2. Twists Luer-lik fittings connecting the bag to the tubing in a counter-clockwise direction and disengages full collection bag.		

3. Replaces full bag with a new collection bag by connecting Luer-lok from new bag to tubing.		
4. Opens side clamps.		
Documentation 1. Records the zero level of the drip chamber on the critical care flow sheet.		
2. Documents nursing assessment of neurological status on critical care flow sheet.		
3. Documents amount of drainage and characteristics q 1° on the critical care flow sheet.		

Self-assessment	Evaluation/ validation methods	Levels	Type of validation	Comments
❑ Experienced ❑ Need practice ❑ Never done ❑ Not applicable (based on scope of practice)	❑ Verbal ❑ Demonstration/ observation ❑ Practical exercise ❑ Interactive class	❑ Beginner ❑ Intermediate ❑ Expert	❑ Orientation ❑ Annual ❑ Other _____	

_______________________________ _______________________________

Employee signature ***Observer signature***

Reference:

Crawford, M. and Drake, J. 2005. Near miss injection of an anesthetic agent into a cerebrospinal fluid external ventricular drain: Special report. *Neurosurgery* 56(5): E116.

Name: ______________________________ Date: ______________

Skill: **Dialysis Fistula Duplex**

Steps	Completed	Comments
1. Check the physician order. Explain the procedure to the patient. Obtain a complete history regarding current and past symptoms. Document surgical procedures.		
2. Assess configuration of graft including type of anastomosis and graft material. Obtain op report if available. Observe graft site for evidence of infection, hematoma, aneurysm. Palpate graft for "thrill."		
3. Image the graft from the arterial anastomosis through the arterial leg, around the loop, and into the venous leg of the graft. Any thrombus formation or sites of increased velocity should be documented with a measurement of peak systolic and % diameter stenosis.		
4. Obtain Doppler velocity waveforms from the arterial inflow vessel; arterial anastomosis; multiple sites throughout the course of the graft; venous anastomosis; and venous outflow vessel using a 60 degree angle.		

5. To determine the flow rate: - Calculate the cross-section area in the transverse view of the venous leg of the graft in an area free of thrombogenic material. Enter on the worksheet. - Obtain a velocity at the same point used for the area with the gate open to sample velocities from the entire lumen. - Press the calc key and cycle through to PI - Cycle to TAMX-trace 3 cardiac cycles and enter. - Multiply this value by 0.5 and enter on worksheet under Mean Velocity. - Calculate the Mean Flow Rate by multiplying the area times the mean velocity. - Multiply this value times 60 to obtain the Mean Flow rate in ml/min and enter on the worksheet. - Videotape and worksheet to physician for interpretation.		

Self-assessment	Evaluation/ validation methods	Levels	Type of validation	Comments
❑ Experienced ❑ Need practice ❑ Never done ❑ Not applicable (based on scope of practice)	❑ Verbal ❑ Demonstration/ observation ❑ Practical exercise ❑ Interactive class	❑ Beginner ❑ Intermediate ❑ Expert	❑ Orientation ❑ Annual ❑ Other _____	

Employee signature

Observer signature

Reference:

Huijbregts, H. et al. 2008. Hemodialysis arteriovenous fistula patency revisited: Results of a prospective, multicenter initiative. *Clinical Journal of the American Society of Nephrology* February 2008.

Name: ______________________________ Date: ______________

Skill: **Discontinuing Esophagogastric Tamponade Tube**

Steps	Completed	Comments
1. Wash hands and don PPE.		
2. Make sure emergency intubation equipment nearby and readily available.		
3. Discontinue in stages to avoid rebleed.		
4. Never deflate gastric balloon while esophageal balloon remains inflated.		
5. Actively deflate esophageal balloon by unclamping the esophageal balloon port and aspirating with an irrigation syringe.		
6. Observe for reoccurrence of bleeding over 24 hours, if bleeding reoccurs, reinflate the gastric balloon.		
7. If no further bleeding noted, deflate gastric balloon after unclamping the gastric balloon port.		
8. Observe for reoccurrence of bleeding over 24 hours, if bleeding reoccurs, reinflate the gastric balloon.		
9. If bleeding has not reoccurred in 24 hours, cut the balloon lumens with scissors and remove tube slowly.		

Self-assessment	Evaluation/ validation methods	Levels	Type of validation	Comments
❑ Experienced ❑ Need practice ❑ Never done ❑ Not applicable (based on scope of practice)	❑ Verbal ❑ Demonstration/ observation ❑ Practical exercise ❑ Interactive class	❑ Beginner ❑ Intermediate ❑ Expert	❑ Orientation ❑ Annual ❑ Other _____	

______________________________ ______________________________

Employee signature *Observer signature*

Reference:

Carlson, K. and Weigand, D. 2005. *AACN procedure manual for critical care.* 5th ed. St. Louis, MO: Elsevier Saunders.

Name: ______________________________ Date: ______________

Skill: **Echocardiogram—Cardiology**

Steps	Completed	Comments
1. Introduces self to patient and explains procedure. Reviews patient data to be certain that the correct test(s) is performed.		
2. Turns machine and tape/disk set on. Selects appropriate preset.		
3. Enters patient information.		
4. Places electrodes on patient.		
5. Positions and instructs patient.		
6. Performs echocardiogram views respectively: • Parasternal long axis • Rv inflow view • Rv out flow views • Parasternal short axis • Av level • Mv level • Lv basal • Lv ppm level • Lv apex • Apical four chamber • Apical two chamber • Apical long axis • Subcostal and suprasternal notch views • Nonstandard views as indicated All views done according to policy/procedure.		
7. Colors with spectral doppler on all patients (must be integrated with each view after anatomic presentation allowing five to 10 cardiac cycles with each view).		
8. Removes electrodes. Cleans gel off patient and transducers and disinfects equipment.		
9. Completes all measurements, paperwork, and log book information accurately.		
10. Delivers patients diagnostic data including folders, tapes, and disks to physician reading station and creates distal folders as indicated.		

Self-assessment	Evaluation/ validation methods	Levels	Type of validation	Comments
❏ Experienced ❏ Need practice ❏ Never done ❏ Not applicable (based on scope of practice)	❏ Verbal ❏ Demonstration/ observation ❏ Practical exercise ❏ Interactive class	❏ Beginner ❏ Intermediate ❏ Expert	❏ Orientation ❏ Annual ❏ Other _____	

_______________________________________ _______________________________________

Employee signature ***Observer signature***

Reference:

Cheitlin, M., et al. 2003. ACC/AHA/ASE 2003 guideline update for the clinical application of echocardiography. *Journal of the American College of Cardiology* September 3, 2003.

Name: ______________________________ Date: ______________

Skill: **EEG—Routine**

Steps	Completed	Comments
1. Identifies self.		
2. Obtains pertinent information from patient history.		
3. Explains procedure to patient: • Electrodes and electrocap • Skin abrasive • Conductors		
4. Demonstrates use of electrocap: • Gloves • Lowering impedance • Gel electrodes		
5. Demonstrates use of EEG machine: • Calibrations with standard settings • Bio Cal • Chooses correct montages and settings • Mark tracing • Activation procedures • Verbalizes minimum guideline standards for recordings • Completes tracing: - Calibrations - Obtains correct data on tracing		
6. Removes electrodes and gel.		
7. Assists patient in combing hair, if necessary.		
8. Returns patient for discharge.		

Self-assessment	Evaluation/ validation methods	Levels	Type of validation	Comments
❑ Experienced ❑ Need practice ❑ Never done ❑ Not applicable (based on scope of practice)	❑ Verbal ❑ Demonstration/ observation ❑ Practical exercise ❑ Interactive class	❑ Beginner ❑ Intermediate ❑ Expert	❑ Orientation ❑ Annual ❑ Other _____	

_______________________________ _______________________________

Employee signature ***Observer signature***

Reference:

American Heart Association. 2005. Guidelines for cardiopulmonary resuscitation and emergency cardiovascular care. *Circulation* 112(Supp. 24): IV1-IV211.

Name: ______________________________ Date: ______________

Skill: **Excel Care ES Bariatric Bed**

Steps	Completed	Comments
1. Demonstrates telescopic vertical height of siderail.		
2. Demonstrate raising/lowering of siderail.		
3. Demonstrates removal and installation of headboard.		
4. Locate drainage bag and patient restraint holders.		
5. Locate footboard caregiver controls and indicators.		
6. Locate enable control key.		
7. Demonstrate raise and lower head and knee sections.		
8. Demonstrate raise and lower bed position.		
9. Demonstrate use of lock-out bed control functions.		
10. Locate "bed not down" indicator.		
11. Locate patient pendant control. Remove and lock in siderail.		
12. Demonstrate head-up/head-down position.		
13. Demonstrate knee-up/knee-down position.		
14. Demonstrate adjusting the width of the bed (all 10 panels).		
15. Demonstrate adjusting length of bed.		
16. Demonstrate use of brake and steer system.		
17. Locate battery backup control. (Stays active for 10 mins after last control operated.)		
18. Locate air supply unit.		
19. Demonstrate removal of air flow unit for access to tight elevator.		
20. Demonstrate patient set-up, height, weight, max inflate and therapy mode.		
21. Demonstrate "fowler boost mode."		
22. Demonstrate lock and unlock of control panel.		

23. Preparing for entry/exit, demonstrate seat inflate/deflate.		
24. Demonstrate deflate and inflate of side bolsters.		
25. Demonstrate deflate and inflate of foot section.		
26. Demonstrate patient transport mode (i.e., side bolster and foot deflation).		
CPR 1. Locate and demonstrate CPR control and Emergency CPR control.		
2. Demonstrate reinflation after CPR.		
Bed Scales 1. Demonstrate zeroing of scale controls.		
2. Demonstrate weighing of the patient.		
3. Locate hold button on scale control. Demonstrate adjusting weight value.		
4. Demonstrate procedure for disconnecting power (pt. in bed) and scale in use.		

Self-assessment	Evaluation/ validation methods	Levels	Type of validation	Comments
❑ Experienced ❑ Need practice ❑ Never done ❑ Not applicable (based on scope of practice)	❑ Verbal ❑ Demonstration/ observation ❑ Practical exercise ❑ Interactive class	❑ Beginner ❑ Intermediate ❑ Expert	❑ Orientation ❑ Annual ❑ Other _____	

_______________________________ _______________________________

Employee signature *Observer signature*

Reference:

Hill-Rom, Inc. 2005. Hill-Rom's new bariatric bed addresses growing obesity trend; designed to safely and comfortably support patients up to 1,000 pounds. *Obesity and Diabetes Week* July 4, 2005.

Name: ______________________________ Date: ______________

Skill: **Femostop Application**

Steps	Completed	Comments
1. Examines puncture site prior to removal of sheath and application of femostop.		
2. Prepares and position femostop belt under and around hips, equally on both sides.		
3. Places center of sterile dome slightly superior and medial to puncture site.		
4. Threads belt through side arm locks and adjusts snugly.		
5. Connects tubing to arch and to manometer; checks tightness of connections to prevent leakage.		
6. Inflates dome to 60 mmHg, dome secured. Inflates dome to 20 mmHg above systolic pressure.		
7. If no bleeding or pulsation observed, maintains pressure at 20 mmHg above systolic pressure and removes arterial sheath.		
8. Gradually reduces compression as follows while assessing for continued hemostasis: a. 20 mmHg above systolic pressure x15 minutes b. 10 mmHg below systolic pressure x15 minutes c. 100 mmHg x30 minutes d. 80 mmHg x30 minutes e. 60 mmHg x30 minutes f. 40 mmHg to complete five hours total of femostop time		
9. Reinflates dome if bleeding/oozing occurs.		
10. Instructs patient on restrictions/complications associated with device per policy.		
11. Removes device and dresses the site per policy.		
12. Documents vital signs, site assessment, and circulation checks every 15 minutes times two, then q 30 min x 4, then every hour until device is removed.		

Self-assessment	Evaluation/ validation methods	Levels	Type of validation	Comments
❏ Experienced ❏ Need practice ❏ Never done ❏ Not applicable (based on scope of practice)	❏ Verbal ❏ Demonstration/ observation ❏ Practical exercise ❏ Interactive class	❏ Beginner ❏ Intermediate ❏ Expert	❏ Orientation ❏ Annual ❏ Other _____	

_______________________________ _______________________________

Employee signature ***Observer signature***

Reference:

Hogg, M. and Kibbe, M. 2006. Percutaneous thoracic and abdominal aortic aneurysm repair: techniques outcomes. *Vascular* 14(5): 270-281.

Name: ______________________________ Date: ______________

Skill: **Hemaquet Removal Postcardiac Catheterization**

Steps	Completed	Comments
1. Observes two sheath removals by RN.		
2. Completes five (minimum) sheath removals independently with RN observing and verbalizes acceptable ACT levels for hemaquet removal.		
3. Gathers equipment : 4x4s, betadine ointment, 5-lb. sandbag, tape.		
4. Wears appropriate PPE: gloves, mask, and shield.		
5. Follows aseptic technique.		
6. Obtains baseline HR, BP, and distal pulse and informs RN prior to removal. Explains procedure.		
7. Has head of bed flat and affected limb straight.		
8. Assesses placement of femoral pulse proximal to insertion site.		
9. Identifies and locates distal pedal and posttibial pulse and grade 1+, 2+, 3+, 4+.		
10. Removes sheath utilizing proper holding technique (notes if sheath is intact).		
11. Maintains manual pressure for a minimum of 10 minutes and observes site for bleeding or hematoma during the hold.		
12. Notifies RN if hematoma develops or if hemostasis is not achieved after 25 minutes.		
13. RN to assess groin prior to application of pressure dressing.		
14. Demonstrates proper dressing application and sandbag placement.		
15. Teaches patient postcatheter instructions and documents.		
16. Verbalizes which catheter should be removed first, when both venous and arterial sheaths are in place.		
17. Completes circulation check of affected limb.		

Self-assessment	Evaluation/ validation methods	Levels	Type of validation	Comments
❑ Experienced ❑ Need practice ❑ Never done ❑ Not applicable (based on scope of practice)	❑ Verbal ❑ Demonstration/ observation ❑ Practical exercise ❑ Interactive class	❑ Beginner ❑ Intermediate ❑ Expert	❑ Orientation ❑ Annual ❑ Other _____	

_______________________________ _______________________________

Employee signature ***Observer signature***

Reference:

Perry, A. and Potter, P. 2006. *Clinical Nursing Skills & Techniques*. 6th ed. St. Louis, MO: Mosby Elsevier.

Name: ______________________________ Date: ______________

Skill: **Identification of Pseudoaneurysm**

Steps	Completed	Comments
1. Palpates pulsatile mass at site of puncture or trauma. a. Does pulse feel broader than artery on opposite limb? b. Does patient complain of localized tenderness? c. Is there ecchymosis of surrounding tissue?		
2. Auscultates mass for presence of bruits.		
3. Assesses extremity distal to mass for circulation.		
4. Contacts physician with findings.		
5. Documents findings and action taken in patient progress notes.		

Self-assessment	Evaluation/ validation methods	Levels	Type of validation	Comments
❑ Experienced ❑ Need practice ❑ Never done ❑ Not applicable (based on scope of practice)	❑ Verbal ❑ Demonstration/ observation ❑ Practical exercise ❑ Interactive class	❑ Beginner ❑ Intermediate ❑ Expert	❑ Orientation ❑ Annual ❑ Other _____	

Employee signature

Observer signature

Reference:

Lough, M., Stacy, K., and Urden, L. 2006. *Thelan's Critical Care Nursing: Diagnosis and Management*. 5th ed. St Louis, MO: Mosby Elsevier.

Name: ______________________________ Date: ______________

Skill: **Lead Placement for Stress Testing**

Steps	Completed	Comments
1. Identifies patient.		
2. Explains procedure to patient.		
3. Shaves patient if applicable, prepares electrode sites with brisk rubbing or sandpaper prep.		
4. Places 10 EKG electrodes according to American Heart Association guidelines: • Right and left upper limb leads just below clavicles. • Right and left lower limb leads adjacent to hips on lower abdomen. • V1 fourth intercostal space right midsternal border. • V2 fourth intercostal space left midsternal border (modify one intercostal space up for SE and DSEs). • V3 halfway between V2 and V4. • V4 fifth intercostal space left midclavicular line. • V5 fifth intercostal space left anterior axillary line. • V6 fifth intercostal space left midaxillary line. (Note: modify V3-V6 down one intercostal space for stress echocardiogram and dobutamine stress echocardiogram.)		

Self-assessment	Evaluation/ validation methods	Levels	Type of validation	Comments
❑ Experienced ❑ Need practice ❑ Never done ❑ Not applicable (based on scope of practice)	❑ Verbal ❑ Demonstration/ observation ❑ Practical exercise ❑ Interactive class	❑ Beginner ❑ Intermediate ❑ Expert	❑ Orientation ❑ Annual ❑ Other _____	

______________________________ ______________________________

Employee signature *Observer signature*

Reference:

Aehlert, B. 2006. *Pocket Reference for ECGs Made Easy.* 3rd ed. St. Louis, MO: Mosby Elsevier.

Name: ______________________________ Date: ______________

Skill: **Mechanical Ventilation**

Steps	Completed	Comments
A. Differentiates volume-cycled modes and pressure -cycled modes		
B. Identifies patient's Mode of Ventilation and adjuncts.		
C. Identifies and documents Ventilator Settings. Tidal volume, Respiratory rate, Mode, F_1O_2, PEEP, PSV, and patient's to response to Mechanical ventilation.		
D. Describes ventilator alarms and their management 1. High pressure alarm (Patient vs. ventilator triggered) 2. Low pressure alarm (Patient vs. ventilator triggered)		
E. Identifies weaning parameters and relationship to ability to wean 1. F_1O_2, ABG, NIF, Respiratory rate, level of consciousness		

Self-assessment	Evaluation/ validation methods	Levels	Type of validation	Comments
❑ Experienced ❑ Need practice ❑ Never done ❑ Not applicable (based on scope of practice)	❑ Verbal ❑ Demonstration/ observation ❑ Practical exercise ❑ Interactive class	❑ Beginner ❑ Intermediate ❑ Expert	❑ Orientation ❑ Annual ❑ Other _____	

Employee signature

Observer signature

Reference:

Berenholtz, S, Milanovich, S, et al. 2004. Improving care for the ventilated patient. *Journal of Quality and Safety* 30(4): 195-204.

Crunden, E., Boyce, C., et al. 2005. An evaluation of the impact of the ventilator care bundle. *Nursing Critical Care* 10(5): 242-246.

Name: ______________________________ Date: ______________

Skill: **Medtronic Pulse Generator**

Steps	Completed	Comments
1. Confirms order for mode and rate.		
2. Replaces battery.		
3. Attaches atrial/ventricular cable(s) to pacer box.		
4. Attaches cable(s) to external pacing wires using procedure gloves.		
5. Verbalizes rational for use of gloves when working with external pacing wires.		
6. Verbalizes indications for use.		
7. Turns pacer on and sets to prescribed mode and rate.		
8. Recognizes/distinguishes a. Failure to sense b. Failure to capture c. Failure to fire Makes appropriate pacer changes.		
9. Saves settings and turns pacer off.		
10. Turns pacer on at saved settings.		
11. Documents date, time of initiation as well as mode, rate, output, and sensitivity.		
12. Obtains and interprets rhythm strip on record.		

Self-assessment	Evaluation/ validation methods	Levels	Type of validation	Comments
❑ Experienced ❑ Need practice ❑ Never done ❑ Not applicable (based on scope of practice)	❑ Verbal ❑ Demonstration/ observation ❑ Practical exercise ❑ Interactive class	❑ Beginner ❑ Intermediate ❑ Expert	❑ Orientation ❑ Annual ❑ Other _____	

______________________________ ______________________________

Employee signature *Observer signature*

Reference:

Del Monte, L., Gamrath, B., and Richards, K. Noninvasive pacing: What you should know. *Journal of Emergency Nursing* 24(3): 223-232.

Name: ______________________________ Date: ______________

Skill: **Miami J® Cervical Collar**

Steps	Completed	Comments
1. Determines collar size.		
2. Takes equipment to bedside and explains procedure to patient/family.		
3. To change from temporary collar: 1. Correctly positions patient.		
2. RN #1 stabilizes patient's neck.		
3. RN #2 loosens Velcro and slides back portion of collar off patient.		Front of collar remains in place.
4. RN #2 slides back of Miami J® collar into position under patient's neck.		Arrows up, centered.
5. RN #2 removes front of temporary collar and places front of Miami J®		Slides it up chest & scoops it under chin off trapezius and toward ears.
6. RN #2 secure Velcro straps one side at a time while assuring no pressure on carotids.		Oriented blue-on-blue to front adhesive. Can stick finger between collar and neck.
7. RN #2 verbalizes criteria for correct fit and what to do if criteria not met.		No pressure on carotids, unable to slide chin. Remove one or both sections & replace with appropriate size. (May be different sizes).

Self-assessment	Evaluation/ validation methods	Levels	Type of validation	Comments
❑ Experienced ❑ Need practice ❑ Never done ❑ Not applicable (based on scope of practice)	❑ Verbal ❑ Demonstration/ observation ❑ Practical exercise ❑ Interactive class	❑ Beginner ❑ Intermediate ❑ Expert	❑ Orientation ❑ Annual ❑ Other _____	

_______________________________ _______________________________

Employee signature *Observer signature*

Reference:

Alspach, J. 2006. *Core Curriculum for Critical Care Nursing*. 6th ed. Saunders.

Name: ______________________ Date: ______________

Skill: **Nasopharyngeal/Tracheal Suctioning**

Steps	Completed	Comments
1. Introduces self.		
2. Explains procedure.		
3. Ensures privacy.		
4. Washes hands.		
5. Assembles equipment.		
6. Positions patient in semi-or-high Fowler's position.		
7. Auscultates lung sounds.		
8. Turns on wall suction.		
9. Opens N/S.		
10. Opens suction catheter kit.		
11. Squeezes lubricant onto sterile field.		
12. Puts on sterile gloves.		
13. Pours N/S.		
14. Attaches catheter to suction tubing.		
15. Draws N/S through catheter.		
16. Lubricates catheter with nondominate hand.		
17. Preoxygenates patient.		
18. Advances catheter into pharynx.		
19. Advances catheter into tracheobronchial tree: a. Advances 2.5-5 cm with inspiration.		
20. Applies intermittent suction by occluding air vent with thumb and drawing catheter in a rotation/twisting monition no longer than 15 seconds.		
21. Flushes catheter tubing with N/S.		
22. Repeats steps 17, 18, 19, and 20, as necessary.		
23. Postoxygenates patient.		
24. Wraps catheter in glove.		

25. Disposes in red trash bags.		
26. Turns off wall suction.		
27. Auscultates lung sounds.		
28. Disposes of supplies.		
29. Documents procedures and sputum characteristics in nurse's notes.		

Self-assessment	Evaluation/ validation methods	Levels	Type of validation	Comments
❑ Experienced ❑ Need practice ❑ Never done ❑ Not applicable (based on scope of practice)	❑ Verbal ❑ Demonstration/ observation ❑ Practical exercise ❑ Interactive class	❑ Beginner ❑ Intermediate ❑ Expert	❑ Orientation ❑ Annual ❑ Other _____	

_______________________________ *Employee signature*

_______________________________ *Observer signature*

Reference:

Perry, A. and Potter, P. 2006. *Clinical Nursing Skills & Techniques.* 6th ed. St. Louis, MO: Mosby Elsevier.

Name: ______________________ Date: ______________

Skill: **Neurologic Examination**

Steps	Completed	Comments
1. Determines orientation to person, place, and time.		
2. Verbalizes cranial nerve being checked and expected response when: a. Using penlight, examines pupils for size, symmetry and reactivity (CN II) b. Checks ocular movement (CN III, IV, VI) c. Instructs patient to raise eyebrows, squeeze eyes shut then open, smile (CN V, VII) d. Instructs patient to stick out tongue, say "Ahh" then put tongue into both cheeks (CN IX, X, XII) e. Instructs patient to shrug shoulders (CN XI)		
3. Recognizes ability to follow directions indicates CN VIII is intact.		
4. Performs sensory checks by touching both sides of patient's forehead, cheek, chin, and lateral and medial surfaces of arms and legs.		
5. Checks motor pathways for symmetry a. Patient to squeeze with each hand b. Patient to perform plantar pushes		
6. Checks for ability to hold arms out to side with palms up and notes presence/absence of "drift"		
7. Stimulates sole of foot from heel to toe and notes Toes Up or Toes Down response.		
8. Documents findings.		
9. Contacts physician in timely manner.		

Self-assessment	Evaluation/ validation methods	Levels	Type of validation	Comments
❑ Experienced ❑ Need practice ❑ Never done ❑ Not applicable (based on scope of practice)	❑ Verbal ❑ Demonstration/ observation ❑ Practical exercise ❑ Interactive class	❑ Beginner ❑ Intermediate ❑ Expert	❑ Orientation ❑ Annual ❑ Other _____	

_______________________ _______________________

Employee signature *Observer signature*

Reference:

Barker, E. 2002. *Neuroscience Nursing: A Spectrum of Care.* 2nd ed. Philadelphia, PA: Mosby.

Name: ______________________________ Date: ______________

Skill: **Preparing for Intubation**

Steps	Completed	Comments
1. Assesses the patient. A = Airway, B = Breathing, C = Circulation		
2. Determines urgency of situation; calls a team (757) or a silent team (calls ICU 53323, pages respiratory therapist 24-9041, and unit manger/ adm. supervisor).		
3. Gathers equipment: • Emergency cart • Intubation box • Suction • Medications • Continuous pulse oximetry • Stethoscope		
4. Explains procedure to patient/family.		
5. Prepares laryngoscope with wither curved or straight blade (per physician's preference).		
6. Prepares ET tube • Opens tube and lubricates • Inserts stylette into ET tube (per physician's preference)		
7. Assists physician with intubation as needed: • Suction • O^2 monitor • Calls out pulse oximeter readings • Administers cricoid pressure if asked • Administers medications as needed • Auscultates breath sounds after intubation		
8. Bags patient after intubation (keep oxygen set at 100%).		
9. Prepares for transfer to critical care unit/OR.		
10. Arranges for further ventilatory support/ventilator.		
11. Reassesses adequacy of ventilation.		

12. Documents procedure including: • Education provided • Who performed the procedure, tube size, meds. • Patient tolerance • Any complications • Patient outcome		

Self-assessment	Evaluation/ validation methods	Levels	Type of validation	Comments
❏ Experienced ❏ Need practice ❏ Never done ❏ Not applicable (based on scope of practice)	❏ Verbal ❏ Demonstration/ observation ❏ Practical exercise ❏ Interactive class	❏ Beginner ❏ Intermediate ❏ Expert	❏ Orientation ❏ Annual ❏ Other _____	

______________________________ ______________________________

Employee signature ***Observer signature***

Reference:
Duell, D., Martin, B., and Smith, S. 2008. *Clinical Nursing Skills: Basic to Advanced Skills*. 7th ed. Upper Saddle River, NJ: Pearson Education, Inc.

Name: ______________________________ Date: ______________

Skill: **Pulmonary Artery Pressure Catheter**

Steps	Completed	Comments
A. Pulmonary artery catheter set-up		
1. Utilizes principle of BSI.		
2. Assembles equipment and pressure line appropriately including: • Connects pressure tubing to flush bag. • Labels flush bag and tubing with date, time, and initials. • Flushes tubing/stopcocks to remove all air from system. • Replaces vented white caps with blue dead-ender caps. • Sets pressure infuser at 300 mmHg. (All the above may be completed by LPN.)		
3. Connects pressure line transducer to monitor.		
4. Connects line to PA catheter, flushes lumens.		
5. Zeros the transducer system prior to insertion of PA catheter and after insertion in pulmonary artery, at level of right atrium.		
6. Inflates balloon for PAWP measurement. Obtains measures at end-expiration.		
7. Obtains PAP and CVP readings at end-expiration.		
8. Documents right atrial, right ventricular, pulmonary artery, and PCWP waveforms and pressure readings during insertion.		
B. PCWP determination		
1. Unlocks balloon inflation valve.		
2. Inflates balloon with minimal amount of air needed to obtain wedging waveform.		
3. PCWP on end-expiration.		
4. Allows balloon to passively deflate.		
5. Relocks balloon inflation valve.		
C. Cardiac output determination		
1. Prepares cardiac output line. Removes all air from bag and line.		

2. Connects cardiac output temperature probe to CO set-up.		
3. Connects cardiac output and thermister cables to monitor.		
4. Prepares syringe/align stopcocks.		
5. Presses start cardiac output. Note: Ready message changed to inject.		
6. Injects 10 ml via Proximal injectate (blue tail) over four seconds. Note: Curve and value.		
7. Repeats (x4), edits, stores.		
8. Resumes IV or pressurized infusion via proximal port (blue tail).		
9. Describes documentation on nurse's progress notes: CO/SVR/CI and amount of air needed to inflate balloon.		
D. Monitoring and maintenance of pulmonary artery catheter		
1. Assesses PAP waveform and documents reading Q 1 h.		
2. Obtains PCWP and cardiac parameters (CO/CI, CVP, SVR) Q 4 hrs or as ordered and documents in nurses notes.		
3. Obtains readings on end-expiration.		
4. Keeps transducer at level of phlebostatic axis at all times (may be performed by LPN).		
5. Changes occlusive dressing Q 72 hours (may be performed by LPN).		
6. Changes pressurized solution and tubings Q 72 hrs. (LPNs may not change tubing once attached to patient.)		
7. Mounts PAP waveform Q shift.		
E. Removal of PA catheter		
1. Utilizes principles of BSI.		
2. Prepares patient • Head position		
3. Assesses site.		

4. Loosens sleeve from introducer and catheter. Note: Paceport-physician must remove pacing wires.		
5. Cleanses site and sutures with povidone iodine.		
6. Turns off appropriate IVs and alarms.		
7. Verifies balloon deflation and removes syringe.		
8. Removes sutures (introducer and PA catheter removal v. PA catheter removal only).		
9. Observes monitor while removing catheter; smoothly pulls catheter through the introducer.		
10. Applies slight pressure over site with 4x4 while removing introducer; apply manual pressure to site x5 minutes (minimum) or until bleeding stops; applies DSD.		
11. Assesses catheter/introducer integrity upon removal/culture tip(s) if appropriate.		
12. If maintaining introducer for continuous infusion, seals end of introducer with sterile obturator and infuses fluids via side port as ordered.		

Self-assessment	Evaluation/ validation methods	Levels	Type of validation	Comments
❑ Experienced ❑ Need practice ❑ Never done ❑ Not applicable (based on scope of practice)	❑ Verbal ❑ Demonstration/ observation ❑ Practical exercise ❑ Interactive class	❑ Beginner ❑ Intermediate ❑ Expert	❑ Orientation ❑ Annual ❑ Other _____	

_______________________________ _______________________________

Employee signature ***Observer signature***

Reference:

Carlson, K. and Weigand, D. 2005. *AACN Procedure Manual for Critical Care*. 5th ed. St. Louis, MO: Elsevier Saunders. 94-95, 476-480, and 579-589.

Name: ______________________________ Date: ______________

Skill: **Spinal Cord Monitoring**

Steps	Completed	Comments
1. Communicates effectively with anesthesia, surgeon, and surgical team.		
2. Obtains pertinent information from patient history.		
3. Establishes protocols regarding recording techniques and levels of anesthesia for each case.		
4. Explains procedure to patient: • Attachment of equipment. • Preparation of equipment.		
5. Identifies electrode impendance and demonstrates adequate troubleshooting techniques.		
6. Demonstrates use of spinal cord monitoring equipment: • Sets up files and trend plots. • Chooses correct recording techniques and settings. • Marks wave forms. • Gathers vitals and anesthesia levels. • Communicates with surgeon and surgical team. • Obtains correct data and documents accurate interpretation of findings.		
7. Removes electrodes.		
8. Demonstrates proper handling and disposal of needles.		
9. Demonstrates proper cleaning technique of equipment.		

Self-assessment	Evaluation/ validation methods	Levels	Type of validation	Comments
❑ Experienced ❑ Need practice ❑ Never done ❑ Not applicable (based on scope of practice)	❑ Verbal ❑ Demonstration/ observation ❑ Practical exercise ❑ Interactive class	❑ Beginner ❑ Intermediate ❑ Expert	❑ Orientation ❑ Annual ❑ Other _____	

______________________________ ______________________________

Employee signature *Observer signature*

Reference:

Alspach, J. (ed.) 2006. *Core curriculum for critical care nursing.* 6th ed. St. Louis, MO: Saunders Elservier.

Name: ______________________________ Date: ______________

Skill: **Thrombolytic Therapy**

Steps	Completed	Comments
Before therapy is begun: 1. Establishes 2 vascular access sites (one may be HL) and checks sites at least q 15 min.		
2. Verbalizes contraindications. (Uncontrolled hypertension, history of bleeding ulcer, active internal bleeding, recent intracranial/intraspinal surgery or trauma, intracranial neoplasm, AV malformation, aneurysm.)		
3. Uses caution/gentleness when moving patient.		
4. Obtains baseline VS and neuron status.		
5. Obtains baseline laboratory values (hemogram, PT, PTT, fibrinogen, electrolytes, CPK).		
6. Avoids repeated needle punctures (blood draws are grouped, avoid IM injections if possible.		
During therapy infusion: 1. Monitor VS and neuron status q 15 min and notifies physician of change immediately.		
2. Checks arm under blood pressure cuff for ecchymosis q 1 hour. Rotates cuff prn.		
3. Monitor for signs of reperfusion (decreased chest pain, resolution of ST elevation, development of arrhythmias).		
4. Looks for subtle signs of bleeding (tachycardia, orthostatic hypotension).		
5. Assess all body drainage for presence of blood and record findings (urine/stool/emesis/gastric drainage).		
6. Monitors lab values (H&H, PT, PTT, other coag, BUN, Creat, Cardiac markers).		
7. Applies pressure to all venipuncture sites for at least 5 minutes.		
8. Identifies risk factors for clot formation (elderly, diabetic, smoking hx., elevated lipids, hypertension, sedentary lifestyle).		

After therapy is completed: 1. Monitors VS and neuron check's q 15 min x 2 hr then q 1 hr x 2 then q 2 hr x 24 hrs.		
2. Monitors lab values using 2nd IV site q 12 h x 24 h then qd x 2.		
3. Assess for subtle signs of bleeding (as above) q 12 h.		
4. Assess for signs of reocclusion and notifies physician immediately (recurrent chest pain, ST segment elevation, diaphoresis, nausea, arrhythmia)		
5. Educates the patient about the current therapy and also the probable use of a " blood thinner" at home (Coumadin booklet).		

Self-assessment	Evaluation/ validation methods	Levels	Type of validation	Comments
❑ Experienced ❑ Need practice ❑ Never done ❑ Not applicable (based on scope of practice)	❑ Verbal ❑ Demonstration/ observation ❑ Practical exercise ❑ Interactive class	❑ Beginner ❑ Intermediate ❑ Expert	❑ Orientation ❑ Annual ❑ Other _____	

Employee signature

Observer signature

Reference:

American College of Cardiology and the American Heart Association. 2004. *ACC/AHA Guideline for the Management of Patients With ST-Elevation Myocardial Infarction Pocket Guide.*

Name: ______________________________ Date: ______________

Skill: **Ventricular Drain**

Steps	Completed	Comments
1. Identify appropriate roles of the RN and LPN a. RN sets up and maintains CSF drainage system b. LPN monitors dressing and system to assure proper working of system c. RN and LPN record and verify amount of drainage per shift		
2. The physician must order the height of the drainage system above or below the zero reference point. Measure the appropriate level of the drainage bag.		
3. If the system malfunctions, notify the physician immediately.		
4. Clamp the VP shunt as per physician's order when removing patient from bed. a. Close roller clamp on tubing before getting patient out of bed. b. Return patient to bed and position drainage bag as the ordered level and unclamp.		
5. Notify the physician immediately if symptoms of increased intracranial pressure, change in mental status, undue loss of fluid, or redness or drainage at the skin site occurs.		
6. Notify the physician if the draining system is cracked, malfunctioning, or damaged, or needs to be changed.		
Positioning of the Drainage Bag 1. Identify the physician order for the drainage bag.		
2. The zero mark on the bag must be hung at the ordered level above or below the VP shunt insertion site. Use measuring tape or laser pointers to determine the level. (Place tape on bag to draw line for each shift level.)		
3. Secure the drainage bag by tying the drainage bag to the IV pole with umbilical or twill tape, plus tape with adhesive.		

4. Any change in the patient's position requires adjustment of the drainage bag to the ordered level.		
5. Check the emptying port on the bag (if set-up has port) for sterile catheter plug, secure with tape as needed.		
General Care 1. Explain to the patient and family that any change in patient's position requires help from the nursing staff to adjust the bag level.		
2. Post a sign over the bed to address activity "Before repositioning this patient, please consult nursing staff."		
3. Chart and mark the approximate amount of ventricular fluid drained each shift and record the amount.		
4. Empty the bag and measure the contents q am (0600). Record on I&O as an actual measurement. It set-up does not have drainage port with plug, change the entire bag.		
Emptying the Drainage Bag Using the Closed System 1. Wash hands; remove tape on catheter plug. Clamp two clamps on tubing.		
2. Measure CSF in clean measuring container or syringe.		
3. Document exact amount on I&O for 24 hours.		
Accidental Disconnection of the VP Drain 1. Call the resident immediately.		
2. Clamp with rubber hemostat until physician is available.		
3. Do not clamp for more than 2 hours without physician approval.		
Documentation 1. Record the zero level of the collection bag and changes required by moving the patient on the Interdisciplinary Plan of Care.		
2. Document nursing observations of level of consciousness on the neurovascular flow sheet.		

3. Document ventricular fluid estimated each shift on the I&O and document actual fluid measurement on the I&O daily.		
4. Document all patient/family teaching related to the VP drain.		

Self-assessment	Evaluation/ validation methods	Levels	Type of validation	Comments
❑ Experienced ❑ Need practice ❑ Never done ❑ Not applicable (based on scope of practice)	❑ Verbal ❑ Demonstration/ observation ❑ Practical exercise ❑ Interactive class	❑ Beginner ❑ Intermediate ❑ Expert	❑ Orientation ❑ Annual ❑ Other _____	

______________________________ ______________________________

Employee signature *Observer signature*

Reference:

Carlson, K. and Weigand, D. 2005. *AACN Procedure Manual for Critical Care*. 5th ed. St. Louis, MO: Elsevier Saunders.

Name: ______________________________ Date: ______________

Skill: **Versacare Bed**

Steps	Completed	Comments
General Features/Functions 1. Demonstrates head-up/down.		
2. Demonstrates auto contour from patient siderail.		
3. Identifies head angle indicator.		
4. Demonstrates knee-up/down.		
5. Demonstrates hi/low.		
6. Demonstrates use of central brake and steer.		
7. Demonstrates use of instant CPR release.		
8. Demonstrates Trendelenburg in a STAT situation.		
9. Demonstrates use of enable key.		
10. Identifies two different ways a patient can move themselves up in bed.		
11. Identifies "Bed Not Down" indicators.		
12. Demonstrates use of easy-grip positioning handles.		
13. Demonstrates how to retract feet and when you use it.		
14. Demonstrates "Auto Firm" and when it's indicated.		
15. Demonstrates Trendelenburg and how to get back in normal position.		
16. Demonstrates foot pedals.		
17. Explains two different ways that bed can help egress patient.		
Patient Position Monitor (PPM) 1. Demonstrates patient position monitor (PPM on/off).		
2. Demonstrates "Position mode."		
3. Demonstrates "Exiting mode."		
4. Demonstrates "Out of bed mode."		
5. Demonstrates volume change.		
6. Demonstrates tone change.		
7. Demonstrates cancel/reset of alarm.		

Patient Pendant 1. Demonstrates how to utilize the pendant.		
2. Demonstrates select control.		
3. Demonstrates use of volume up/down.		
Lockout Features 1. Identifies head siderail, knee siderail, hi/low and all motor features.		
Bed Scale 1. Identifies how to zero the scale and what the scale should be zeroed with (per practice).		
2. Demonstrates how to turn scale on/off.		
3. Demonstrates how to properly weigh a patient.		
Miscellaneous Features 1. Demonstrates low chair position.		
2. Identifies Battery Back-up and how to activate it.		
3. Identifies head up angle indicator.		
4. Identify trend angle indicator.		
5. Identifies automatic night light.		
6. Demonstrates headboard removal.		
7. Demonstrates IV pole placement.		
8. Identifies restraint strap holders.		
9. Demonstrates IV pole storage.		
10. Discusses siderail pads.		
11. Discusses traction.		
12. Demonstrates pendant controls.		
13. Demonstrates moving/steering bed.		

Self-assessment	Evaluation/ validation methods	Levels	Type of validation	Comments
❑ Experienced ❑ Need practice ❑ Never done ❑ Not applicable (based on scope of practice)	❑ Verbal ❑ Demonstration/ observation ❑ Practical exercise ❑ Interactive class	❑ Beginner ❑ Intermediate ❑ Expert	❑ Orientation ❑ Annual ❑ Other _____	

Employee signature

Observer signature

Reference:

Bell-Syer, S., et al. 2004. Support surfaces for pressure ulcer prevention. *Cochrane Database of Systematic Reviews* 3: CD001735.

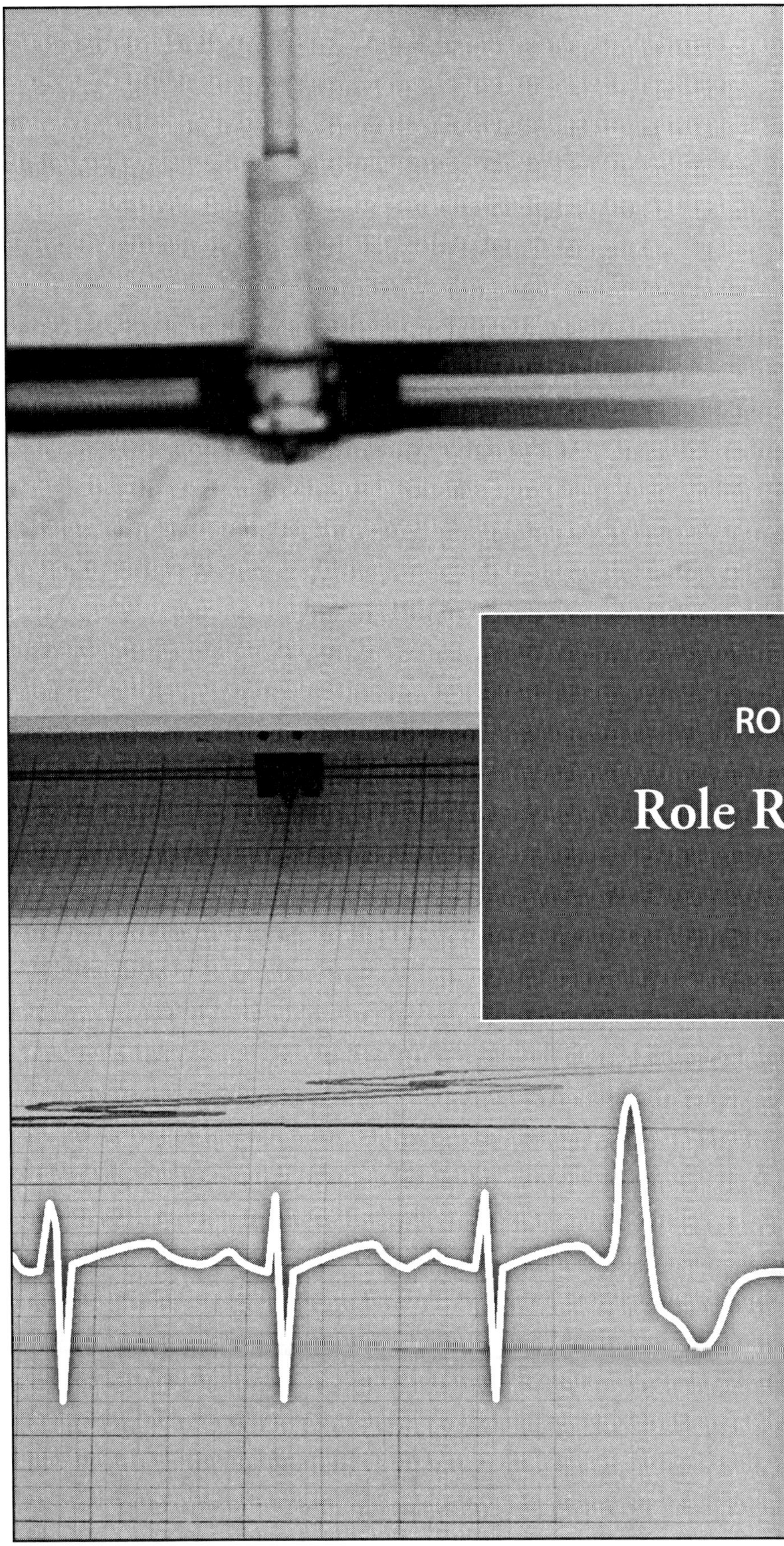

ROLE

Role Related

Contents

Name: ______________________________ Date: ______________

Skill: **Acid Mixing**

Steps	Completed	Comments
1. Rinses tank (only if changing type of acid). Rinses tank: • Sprays inside of tank with hose. • Opens water valve (red valve on side of vat) and add some water. • Opens manual drain briefly. • Opens drain valve and turn on transfer pump to drain remaining fluid. • Turns off transfer pump.		
2. Obtains appropriate acid supply boxes (2 or 3k). Fills tank to 15–20 gallons and then adds liquid mix. Always add liquid first.		
3. Turns bicarb mixer 2 on and then adds dry powder: red, green, then white bags. Always in that order.		
4. Turns mixer off when tank gets close to two-gallon mark. Turns off water supply to tank when level reaches 25 gallons.		
5. Turns mixer back on and runs until it automatically shuts off (approximately 10 minutes).		
6. Is certain which acid was mixed (2k or 3k) and puts label on vat.		
7. Opens proper valve (2k or 3k). (All other valves should be closed.)		
8. Turns off transfer pump, watches level in the tank, and turns off transfer pump when tank is empty.		

Self-assessment	Evaluation/ validation methods	Levels	Type of validation	Comments
❑ Experienced ❑ Need practice ❑ Never done ❑ Not applicable (based on scope of practice)	❑ Verbal ❑ Demonstration/ observation ❑ Practical exercise ❑ Interactive class	❑ Beginner	❑ Orientation ❑ Annual ❑ Other _____	

Employee signature ______________________ Observer signature ______________________

Name: ______________________________ Date: ______________

Skill: **Adding Toner to Fax**

Steps	Completed	Comments
1. Watch for "add toner" light.		
2. Open cartridge cover by pulling the lever above the arrow mark.		
3. Remove the old cartridge.		
4. Remove a new cartridge from the protective bag.		
5. Rock the new cartridge five or six times to distribute the toner evenly inside the cartridge.		
6. Place the cartridge on a flat, clean surface.		
7. Steady the cartridge with one hand and remove the seal by gently pulling on the plastic tab with your other hand.		
8. Load the cartridge in the direction indicated by the arrow.		
9. Gently slide the cartridge into the printer until it is down inside the main unit and level.		
10. Close the cartridge cover.		

Self-assessment	Evaluation/ validation methods	Levels	Type of validation	Comments
❑ Experienced ❑ Need practice ❑ Never done ❑ Not applicable (based on scope of practice)	❑ Verbal ❑ Demonstration/ observation ❑ Practical exercise ❑ Interactive class	❑ Beginner ❑ Intermediate ❑ Expert	❑ Orientation ❑ Annual ❑ Other _____	

______________________________ ______________________________

Employee signature *Observer signature*

Name: ______________________________ Date: ______________

Skill: **Administrative Associate Accurate Charging**

Steps	Completed	Comments
1. Demonstrates accurate charging with the following items:		
a. Apnea management		
b. Exchange transfusion		
c. Resuscitation		
d. IV insertion		
e. Cascade set-up		
f. Vent set-up		
g. Survanta		
h. Disposable LP tray		
i. Pulse oximeter		
j. Pulse oximeter checks		
k. Neonatal transport (up to one and a half hours)		
l. Neonatal transport (additional half hour)		
m. Circumcision		
n. Cardiac respiratory monitors		
o. Apnea homecare training		
p. Phototherapy		
q. Eye exams		
r. Syringe pump (feeds)		
s. Syringe pump (meds)		
t. Disposable BP cuffs		
2. Batches items and sends to data processing.		

Self-assessment	Evaluation/ validation methods	Levels	Type of validation	Comments
❑ Experienced ❑ Need practice ❑ Never done ❑ Not applicable (based on scope of practice)	❑ Verbal ❑ Demonstration/ observation ❑ Practical exercise ❑ Interactive class	❑ Beginner ❑ Intermediate ❑ Expert	❑ Orientation ❑ Annual ❑ Other ______	

______________________________ ______________________________

Employee signature *Observer signature*

Name: ______________________________ Date: ______________

Skill: **Age-Specific Competency Checklist RN/LPN**

Steps	Completed	Comments
Alters care given on age-specific needs.		
A. Physical		
Adolescent – increases need for nourishment/nutrition.		
Early adulthood – alters diet, decreases amount of food.		
Middle adult – provides assistance with ambulation, provides moisture, keeps temperature set for comfort.		
Late adult – close observation of vital signs, I&O stays alert for drug-drug interactions.		
B. Motor/sensory adaptation		
Adolescent – assists with ambulation, provides for sleep.		
Early adulthood – ensures decreased background noise, encourages use of glasses.		
Middle adult – speaks loudly, assists with ambulation.		
Late adult – does not rush patient; provides glasses, hearing aids for assistance.		
C. Cognitive		
Adolescent – speaks to patient as an adult not a child.		
Early adulthood – identifies learning preferences.		
Middle adult – alters patient education techniques.		
Late adult – encourages participation in society, social groups.		
D. Psychosocial		
Adolescence – encourages peers to visit/phone, explores feelings with patients.		

Early adulthood – explores how illness will stress job, family, and responsibilities.		
Middle adult – helps patient identify stressors and his or her relationship to illness.		
Late adult – assesses patient's place in society, addresses concerns.		

Self-assessment	Evaluation/ validation methods	Levels	Type of validation	Comments
❑ Experienced ❑ Need practice ❑ Never done ❑ Not applicable (based on scope of practice)	❑ Verbal ❑ Demonstration/ observation ❑ Practical exercise ❑ Interactive class	❑ Beginner ❑ Intermediate ❑ Expert	❑ Orientation ❑ Annual ❑ Other _____	

_______________________________   _______________________________

Employee signature   ***Observer signature***

Name: ______________________________ Date: ______________

Skill: **Age-Specific Competency Checklist SA/AA**

Steps	Completed	Comments
Alters care based on age-specific needs.		
A. Physical		
Adolescent – provides snacks.		
Early adulthood – provides alternative foods within diet.		
Middle adult – sets room temperature for patient comfort.		
Late adult – measures urine output, reports changes to nurse.		
B. Motor/sensory adaptation		
Adolescent – assists with ambulation, provides for rest.		
Early adulthood – keeps area quiet.		
Middle adult – speaks slowly, assists with ambulation.		
Late adult – does not rush patient.		
C. Cognitive		
Adolescent – treats patient as an adult.		
Early adulthood – helps patient to alleviate boredom.		
Middle adult – repeats instructions as needed—answers questions.		
Late adult – encourages activities.		
D. Psychosocial		
Adolescent – encourages patient to talk, participate.		
Early adulthood – participates in identification of stress of patient and reports to nurse.		

Middle adult – participates in identification of stressors and reports to nurse.		
Late adult – encourages participant in ADLs—offers to help when needed.		

Self-assessment	Evaluation/ validation methods	Levels	Type of validation	Comments
❑ Experienced ❑ Need practice ❑ Never done ❑ Not applicable (based on scope of practice)	❑ Verbal ❑ Demonstration/ observation ❑ Practical exercise ❑ Interactive class	❑ Beginner ❑ Intermediate ❑ Expert	❑ Orientation ❑ Annual ❑ Other _____	

_______________________________ *Employee signature*

_______________________________ *Observer signature*

Name: ______________________________ Date: ______________

Skill: **Appointment Scheduling—Diabetes Center**

Steps	Completed	Comments
1. Determines accurate spelling of patient's full name on outpatient order form.		
2. Contacts patient for scheduling within one business day after receiving the order.		
3. Notifies physician and diabetes center staff of scheduling problems with a patient.		
4. Schedules correct appointment type with appropriate information given to the patient regarding the appointment and what to bring.		
5. Documents patient's insurance information and refers patient to patient account services when appropriate.		
6. Instructs patient to call his or her insurance company to check on coverage for diabetes education prior to coming to the first appointment.		
7. Obtains approval from the educator for overbooking appointments, based on patient's needs.		

Self-assessment	Evaluation/ validation methods	Levels	Type of validation	Comments
❑ Experienced ❑ Need practice ❑ Never done ❑ Not applicable (based on scope of practice)	❑ Verbal ❑ Demonstration/ observation ❑ Practical exercise ❑ Interactive class	❑ Beginner ❑ Intermediate ❑ Expert	❑ Orientation ❑ Annual ❑ Other _____	

Employee signature

Observer signature

Name: ______________________________ Date: ______________

Skill: **Behavioral Health Associate**

Steps	Completed	Comments
A. Phlebotomy & Advanced Technical Skills:		
1. Veinpuncture procedure		
2. Finger stick procedure		
3. Blood bank procedure		
4. Quality Control procedure		
5. Blood Glucose Testing procedure		
6. Blood pressure		
B. Review: Demonstrates ability to obtain and transport appropriately the following speci-mens:		
1. Sputum		
2. Urine/Routine/CCMS		
3. Stool		
4. Blood		

Self-assessment	Evaluation/ validation methods	Levels	Type of validation	Comments
❑ Experienced ❑ Need practice ❑ Never done ❑ Not applicable (based on scope of practice)	❑ Verbal ❑ Demonstration/ observation ❑ Practical exercise ❑ Interactive class	❑ Beginner ❑ Intermediate ❑ Expert	❑ Orientation ❑ Annual ❑ Other _____	

______________________________ ______________________________

Employee signature *Observer signature*

Name: ______________________________ Date: ______________

Skill: **Bicarb Mixing**

Steps	Completed	Comments
1. Checks that mix tank is empty and clean.		
2. Checks that valve 8D is closed.		
3. Determines batch size to be made, 50 to 100 gallons. (We average 150–200 gal. per day.)		
4. For 100 gal., turns fill to "on" and presses "fill start." When mix tank has filled to 95 gal., marks it (automatically shuts off). (Takes approx. 30 minutes.)		
5. For 50 gal, turns fill to "on" and presses "fill start." When mix tank reaches 45 gal., marks it, turns fill switch to "off."		
6. Opens valve 6M.		
7. Turns mix to "on" and presses "mix start." Add dry chemical to mix tank (one bag per 25 gal.). It will mix for 30 minutes and has auto shut-off.		
8. After mix is complete, checks that all dry chemical has dissolved.		

Self-assessment	Evaluation/ validation methods	Levels	Type of validation	Comments
❑ Experienced ❑ Need practice ❑ Never done ❑ Not applicable (based on scope of practice)	❑ Verbal ❑ Demonstration/ observation ❑ Practical exercise ❑ Interactive class	❑ Beginner ❑ Intermediate ❑ Expert	❑ Orientation ❑ Annual ❑ Other _____	

______________________________ ______________________________

Employee signature *Observer signature*

Name: ______________________________ Date: ______________

Skill: **Charge Entry**

Steps	Completed	Comments
1. User performs entering a charge from start to finish.		
2. Demonstrates changing the date and quality fields.		
3. Explains the ramifications of exiting out of the change screen without using the update button.		
4. Identifies when, why, and how to change an account before entering a charge.		

Self-assessment	Evaluation/ validation methods	Levels	Type of validation	Comments
❑ Experienced ❑ Need practice ❑ Never done ❑ Not applicable (based on scope of practice)	❑ Verbal ❑ Demonstration/ observation ❑ Practical exercise ❑ Interactive class	❑ Beginner ❑ Intermediate ❑ Expert	❑ Orientation ❑ Annual ❑ Other _____	

Employee signature

Observer signature

Name: ______________________________ Date: ______________

Skill: **Charge Nurse Assessment/Evaluation**

Steps	Completed	Comments
A. **Clinical/Technical Competencies:** *Responsibilities directly related to patient care or some technical aspect of working on a clinical unit.* 1. Enter patient acuities into Optilink computer (or ensure these are done) according to policy.		
2. Assist staff in completing their work.		
3. Act as a clinical resource, sharing knowledge.		
4. Use computer skills to chart and complete reports.		
5. Delegate workload appropriately and fairly.		
6. Check emergency equipment handle unit emergencies.		
7. Conducts initial unitwide patient assessments.		
8. Knowledge of medical equipment to provide care.		
9. Knowledgeable of available clinical resources when needed.		
10. Knowledgeable of unit, type of patients, procedures, etc. to plan work.		
11. Maintain a safe, clean physical unit environment.		
12. Provide direct care as needed, balancing patient care with charge nurse duties.		
13. Give an effective change of shift report to oncoming Charge Nurse.		
14. Coordinates shift assignments for all staff and delegates patient care according to patient acuity, assures nursing assistants will be given specific patient care assignments.		
15. Facilitates patient safety.		
B. **Critical Thinking Competencies:** *Responsibilities that address effective decision making and problem solving involving both critical and operational issues on the unit.* 1. Anticipate patient needs, staffing requirements; engage in anticipatory planning and generating solutions.		

2. Assess/evaluate clinical and operational information.		
3. Manage crises as they occur.		
4. Make decisions.		
5. Uses good judgment.		
6. Prioritizes—decides the order of importance of tasks.		
7. Uses knowledge of patient status to plan care.		
8. Uses knowledge of staff capabilities to plan care.		
9. Troubleshoot—problem solve to prevent a potential crisis.		
10. Manage time effectively.		
11. Assess requirements and takes action to provide adequate staff.		
12. Know and deal with personal limitations.		
13. Deal effectively with change.		
C. Organizational Competencies: *Responsibilities to understand and operate in the organizational environment on the unit as well as in the larger institutions (hospital, agency, etc.).* 1. Coordinate multiple tasks in order to keep unit operations flowing.		
2. Deal with interruptions.		
3. Uses a method to keep organized.		
4. Prepare prior to the beginning of shift.		
5. Know and use hospital/unit policies and patient procedures appropriately.		
6. Oversee unit functions to ensure overall quality of care/practice.		
7. Coordinate the following functions:		
a. TTO/Floating under the direction of the Unit Manager/Administrative Supervisor.		
b. The Float nurse's assignment. Acts as a resource to the float nurse.		
c. Relocated staff during emergencies.		
d. Assures completeness of staff partnership assignments sheet.		

8. Reviews staffing patterns for the oncoming shift with the Unit Manager. Assigns nursing assistants to the RN leaders/and partnerships. At shift change (i.e. 3:00pm) the Charge Nurse reviews the assignments for nursing assistants in collaboration with the partnership leaders. Together they determine what remaining tasks need to be completed and delegates these tasks to the oncoming nursing assistant to partnership as needed, in collaboration with the Charge Nurse that is leaving.		
9. Assigns breaks and lunches and marks on board/assignment sheet.		
a. Staff report on and off the unit to the Charge Nurse. The staff documents and/or verbally reports the time they leave and return to the unit on the unit board.		
b. The staff will adhere to their assigned/designated break time.		
10. Assigns beds using telechecking responds in 15 minutes.		
11. Assigns meeting/inservice attendance and coverage as appropriate in collaboration with the Unit Manager or Administrative supervisor.		
12. Reports unusual occurrences, medication errors, on-the-job accidents, patient complaints and visitor illness, injury to Unit Manager/Assistant Unit Manager/Administrative Supervisor.		
13. Monitors the ADT log for accuracy of census in collaboration with the Unit Secretary and in their absence.		
14. Reviews sitter cases in collaboration with the Unit Manager/Patient Care Coordinator every shift. Documents sitter cases on assignment sheet.		
15. Clarifies policy and procedures and/or directs questions to the Unit Manager/Administrative Supervisor.		
16. Understand what is happening in whole hospital in order to adjust running the unit.		
17. Manage cost and supply issues.		

D. Human Relations Skills Competencies: *Responsibilities to interact effectively with other personnel to accomplish the requirements of patient care as well as administrative activities.* 1. Be accessible—identify self as the charge nurse.		
2. Influence atmosphere of unit in positive manner.		
3. Demonstrate caring for others.		
4. Communicate effectively with charge nurse, ongoing/off-going shift, physicians, patient's families, staff, supervisors.		
5. Communicates with the on-coming/off-going charge nurse to convey patient care concerns/needs, staffing issues, and utilizes effective problem-solving skills in the delivery of nursing care.		
6. Communicates concerns to the Unit Manager/Administrative supervisor.		
7. Deals with difficult people, situations, shifts.		
8. Uses diplomacy with people.		
9. Gets along with people.		
10. Interacts positively with nurse manager.		
11. Provides leadership during the shift.		
12. Motivates staff to accomplish the mission.		
13. Protects staff.		
14. Addresses patient complaints, utilizing service recovery plan.		
15. Role-models effectively.		
16. Acts as a resource to the nursing staff (including agency nurses).		
17. Develop and train the staff.		
18. Supports staffs' personal needs.		
19. Team build—develop cooperative efforts.		
20. Assists in the development and maintenance of a supportive unit climate in which staff members respond to each other in a way that contributes to effective team building.		

Self-assessment	Evaluation/ validation methods	Levels	Type of validation	Comments
❑ Experienced ❑ Need practice ❑ Never done ❑ Not applicable (based on scope of practice)	❑ Verbal ❑ Demonstration/ observation ❑ Practical exercise ❑ Interactive class	❑ Beginner ❑ Intermediate ❑ Expert	❑ Orientation ❑ Annual ❑ Other _____	

Employee signature

Observer signature

Name: ______________________________ Date: ________________

Skill: **Defibrillator Function—Daily Check (Lifepak 9)**

Steps	Completed	Comments
1. Verifies paddles are firmly seated in test load (storage) area.		
2. Pushes 2 "energy select." Selects 200 joules if not already selected.		
3. Pushes 3 "charge." "Joules changing" will appear in lower right corner of monitor screen. Increasing numbers indicate energy level as defi brillator charges.		
4. Determines defibrillator is ready when the selected energy and the "joules available" messages appear in the lower right corner of monitor screen.		
5. Ascertains that "charge" button indicator light glows steadily and a charge complete tone is heard. Determines charge cycle takes ≤ 10 seconds.		
6. Pushes the apex discharge button only and verifies the unit does not discharge.		
7. Pushes the sternum discharge button only and verifies that unit does not discharge.		
8. Discharges defibrillator by pushing both paddle discharge buttons simultaneously.		
9. Verifies the message "test 200 joules delivered" appears in lower right corner of screen for three seconds.		
10. Retrieves recorder printout of "time, date, and defib test 200 joules delivered."		
11. Documents on daily log of defibrillator readiness for use.		

Self-assessment	Evaluation/ validation methods	Levels	Type of validation	Comments
❑ Experienced ❑ Need practice ❑ Never done ❑ Not applicable (based on scope of practice)	❑ Verbal ❑ Demonstration/ observation ❑ Practical exercise ❑ Interactive class	❑ Beginner ❑ Intermediate ❑ Expert	❑ Orientation ❑ Annual ❑ Other _____	

______________________________ ______________________________

Employee signature *Observer signature*

Name: ______________________________ Date: ______________

Skill: **Discharge Bed/Bassinette Cleaning for Environmental Associates**

Steps	Completed	Comments
1. Apply gloves. Use goggles if mixing concentrate.		
2. Mix germicidal cleaning solution, diluting concentrate correctly.		
3. Remove the pillow case from the pillow. Set aside. Remove the pillow case from the bassinette mattress.		
4. Carefully loosen the linen from the corners of the bed and roll toward the center of the bed to make a neat bundle. Place the rolled bundle of linen into the pillow case.		
5. Check the bedside table and the patient restroom for any wash cloths and bath towels so that they can be disposed of with the soiled linen.		
6. Wash bassinette.		
7. Wipe the patient's pillow with the cleaning cloth, which has been wrung out in the germicidal solution.		
8. Raise the head and foot of the bed by the remote switch.		
9. Wring out the cleaning cloth in the germicidal solution. Wipe down one half of the headboard, cleaning both front and back.		
10. Move on to wipe on half of the mattress and bed frame. Begin by wiping the top of the mattress.		
11. Wring out cleaning cloth in germicidal solution and wipe the bed frame and bedrails.		
12. For cleaning the footboard, follow the same cleaning procedure used on the headboard.		
13. After cleaning the other side of the mattress, headboard, bed frame, bedrails, and footboard, return the mattress to its normal position.		
14. Empty germicidal solution in restroom toilet.		
15. Get clean linen from linen closet.		
16. Make the bed.		

17. Set up room for next patient.		

Self-assessment	Evaluation/ validation methods	Levels	Type of validation	Comments
❏ Experienced ❏ Need practice ❏ Never done ❏ Not applicable (based on scope of practice)	❏ Verbal ❏ Demonstration/ observation ❏ Practical exercise ❏ Interactive class	❏ Beginner ❏ Intermediate ❏ Expert	❏ Orientation ❏ Annual ❏ Other _____	

_______________________________ _______________________________

Employee signature *Observer signature*

Name: ____________________ Date: ____________

Skill: **HOP Charges**

Steps	Completed	Comments
1. Identifies if patient is a 23 hour assign/HOP/EO or admitted.		
2. Identifies on the HOP patient (includes the patient's written assign or EO) the time the observation expires. At this time (or before this time), alerts the RN to notify the physician of the need for the admit order to be written.		
3. Identifies correct "Hourly Observation Charges form."		
4. Stamps form with the correct patient name plate.		
5. Records the date/time in (arrival time to the unit) and the date/time out (time patient was discharged from the unit, or transferred to ICU, SCVICU, or taken to the OR then admitted to another floor—use time the order was written; if no order written then use the time the patient left the observation floor).		
6. Calculates the difference from the time assigned to the time discharged/admitted. Rounds to the nearest hour (no minutes; i.e., if 1–29 minutes, drops the minute, keeps only the hour; if 30–59 minutes, then round to the next hour).		
7. Places the calculated hour amount in the correct unit line.		
8. Sends the form urgent mail to "data entry at Summa Center." Sends all forms from each unit together every morning.		
9. Delivers to the urgent mail box.		
10. Follows up with a status change form: if being discharged or being changed to an admitted patient, marks form accordingly and faxes to admitting.		

Self-assessment	Evaluation/ validation methods	Levels	Type of validation	Comments
❑ Experienced ❑ Need practice ❑ Never done ❑ Not applicable (based on scope of practice)	❑ Verbal ❑ Demonstration/ observation ❑ Practical exercise ❑ Interactive class	❑ Beginner ❑ Intermediate ❑ Expert	❑ Orientation ❑ Annual ❑ Other _____	

Employee signature

Observer signature

Name: ______________________________ Date: ______________

Skill: **Insurance Precertification Authorization**

Steps	Completed	Comments
1. Examines the chart for type of insurance.		
2. Determines if test needs precertified or authorized.		
3. Calls the phone number on the insurance card for benefits verification and authorization.		
4. Gives insurance company information regarding test ordered.		
5. Documents in chart: • Name of person spoke with at insurance company • Authorization number (if applicable)		
6. Enters authorization number into MPAC INVU screen.		
7. Identifies resource person if difficulties arise.		

Self-assessment	Evaluation/ validation methods	Levels	Type of validation	Comments
❑ Experienced ❑ Need practice ❑ Never done ❑ Not applicable (based on scope of practice)	❑ Verbal ❑ Demonstration/ observation ❑ Practical exercise ❑ Interactive class	❑ Beginner ❑ Intermediate ❑ Expert	❑ Orientation ❑ Annual ❑ Other _____	

______________________________ ______________________________

Employee signature *Observer signature*

Name: ______________________________ Date: ______________

Skill: **LPN Skills Assessment/Evaluation**

Steps	Completed	Comments
I. Competency A. Nursing Process 1. Assists RN in data collection, implementation, and evaluation of nursing care.		
2. Provides patient teaching.		
3. Prioritizes care for a group of patients.		
4. Utilizes appropriate resources.		
B. Technical Skills 1. Monitors/discontinues IVs.		
2. Maintains gastric/feeding tubes.		
3. Inserts/maintains urinary catheters.		
4. Performs trach care and suctioning.		
5. Assesses patient safety including proper utilization of restraints.		
6. Completes tissue therapy.		
7. Completes American Heart Association guidelines for BLS-Healthcare provider in CPR.		
8. Sets oxygen gauge rate.		
9. Locates various items on the emergency cart.		
10. Identifies nursing responsibilities in emergency situations.		
11. Provides and documents pre- and postop nursing care.		
12. Incorporates nursing measures to reduce and prevent the spread of infection in daily nursing care.		
13. Performs neurological checks when appropriate.		
14. Draws blood routine blood specimens.		
15. Performs BGT.		
16. Performs Blood Culture.		
17. Other		

C. Medications 1. Completes medication exam with a minimum score of 80%.		
2. Describes usual dose, common side effects, compatibilities, action, and untoward reactions of medications.		
3. Administers medications a. I.M.		
b. SQ and Insulin		
c. Calculations		
d. Other		
4. Documents administration of medication (MAR, controlled drugs, etc.)		
5. Identifies medication error reporting system.		
II. Accountability/Leadership A. Completes orientation statement of agreement.		
B. Accepts responsibilities as delegated.		
C. Follows appropriate employee policies and procedures, i.e. call off, time off, LOA, etc.		
D. Conforms to dress code.		
E. Identifies role of the nurse in quality assurance.		
F. Maintains safe working environment.		
G. Contains costs through proper use of supplies and maintenance of equipment.		
III. Communication A. Documents on the following forms: Interdisciplinary Assessment		
Graphic Record/PLATO.		
Interdisciplinary Progress Record		
Nursing Ongoing Assessment		
Unusual Occurrence		
B. Uses correct lines of communication.		
C. Attends Computer Class.		
D. Gives prompt, accurate, and pertinent report RN.		
E. Interacts with patients, significant others and health team members in positive manner.		

IV. Other A. Has completed Human Resources/Survey Orientation.		

Self-assessment	Evaluation/ validation methods	Levels	Type of validation	Comments
❑ Experienced ❑ Need practice ❑ Never done ❑ Not applicable (based on scope of practice)	❑ Verbal ❑ Demonstration/ observation ❑ Practical exercise ❑ Interactive class	❑ Beginner ❑ Intermediate ❑ Expert	❑ Orientation ❑ Annual ❑ Other _____	

_______________________________ *Employee signature*

_______________________________ *Observer signature*

Name: ______________________________ Date: ______________

Skill: **Nursing Assistant Orientation Skills Assessment/Evaluation**

Steps	Completed	Comments
A. Ability to do basic patient care as follows: Complete bed bath.		
Partial bath.		
Assists with shower.		
Oral hygiene (bid & prn).		
Back care.		
Peri care.		
Hair care.		
Offering/removal of bed pan or urinal.		
Ambulatory/assist to bathroom.		
Cath care.		
Documentation of output on bedside worksheet.		
Feeding patient, including compensatory strategies for feeding dysphagic patient.		
Assists patient with meeting all basic patient needs, toileting, walking, call light, etc.		
Makes Occupied bed.		
Makes Unoccupied bed.		
Accurately measures patient intake & output and records.		
Patient transfer/discharge.		
Supports safety of patient i.e. side rails, slippers or pt. lift, prn.		
Pneumatic Cuffs: Anti-embolic Therapy applied correctly.		
Uses hot (T-pad) and cold (ice) therapy safely.		
Uses **patient safety** properly, i.e., documentation of restraints.		
B. Communication skills Responds to call lights promptly.		
Anticipates & clarifies needs, i.e. pain, weakness, verbalizes to patient's nurse when needed.		

C. Provide age appropriate care 1. Recognizes need/independent decision-making (adults).		
2. Promotes bowel & bladder continence per toileting schedule.		
3. Provides privacy.		
4. Assist/orientation to room, equipment & surroundings.		
5. Removes dirty linen or equipment from patient room.		
D. Provides nutrition support 1. Passes and picks up trays, setting items up for ease of use.		
2. Records Intake (& output) accurately on worksheet in room.		
3. Identifies the percentage eaten of meals accurately in PLATO.		
4. Positions the patient for safety and comfort prior to eating.		
5. Encourages and assists with patient's meals, being aware of specific needs, and feeding patients as needed.		
E. Technical skills 1. BLS course: Heartsaver or Health Care Provider (optional).		
2. Assures patient's nurse is monitoring oxygen before & after activities (i.e. transport).		
3. Identifies responsibilities in emergency situations.		
4. Uses measures to reduce and prevent spread of infection in daily patient care.		
5. **Demonstrates ability to take and record vital signs** a. Takes **oral &/or axillary Temperature** & records.		
b. Use electronic automated blood pressure machine to take BP & records.		
c. Counts (30 seconds) & records **Radial pulse** rate accurately or records pulse from BP machine.		

d. Counts **respiratory rate** and records accurately.		
e. Reports variances, and patient needs to patient's Nurse for follow-up.		
F. <u>Demonstrates ability to obtain and transport specimens</u> 1. Sputum		
2. Urine/routine & CCMS		
3. Stool		
G. <u>Body mechanics</u> 1. Demonstrates proper lifting/turning/transferring patient techniques.		
2. Demonstrates proper technique in transferring patient from bed to cart and back.		
3. Uses proper positions & turning, protecting skin & bony prominences. Uses turning schedule.		
H. <u>Environmental needs</u> 1. Replaces trash bags, removes excess linen, etc. from rooms.		
2. Keeps pathways clear, free from clutter, checks lights, & other equipment in patient room.		
I. <u>Performs postmortem care</u>		
J. <u>Assists with transport of patient to the morgue</u>		
K. <u>Safety</u> 1. Verbalizes safety issues with equipment (step ladders, hand tools, light bulbs, etc.) to patient's nurse.		
2. Reports problems with lighting, equipment or supplies that cannot be repaired by nursing staff to maintenance.		
3. Identifies light maintenance duties.		
L. Demonstrates ability to **<u>Contact Distribution</u>** Department for needed patient care items.		
M. <u>Unit Communication</u> 1. Documents on patient chart on Nursing Treatment Record & PLATO accurately		
2. Telephone/answers phone by identifying unit, name, & status.		

3. Operates pneumatic tube system/describes use (Class)		
4. Uses principles of patient confidentiality.		
5. Communicating to RN – any unusual observations (Signs and Symptoms) **PROMPTLY**.		
N. Interacts positively with patients, their significant others, and health team members.		
O. Punctuality 1. Arrives promptly in uniform.		
2. Notifies nursing office of absences by nursing policy.		
3. Notifies nursing office of lateness per policy.		
4. Notifies nurse in charge if leaving unit, returns promptly.		
P. Safety issues (Should be able to discuss and correctly answer questions on the following safety topics) 1. Fire Safety (Code Red)		
2. Bomb Threat (Code Black)		
3. Code Blue (Medical)		
4. Code Violet		
5. Infection Prevention & Exposure Control		
6. Disaster (Code Yellow)		
7. Evacuation		
8. Back Safety		
9. Severe Weather		
10. Electrical Safety		
11. Code Adam		
Q. Examinations 1. Standard precautions & Terminology		
2. Patient Safety		
3. Patient Limited Activity		
4. Hygiene		
R. SLPs		
S. Unit Competencies		

Self-assessment	Evaluation/ validation methods	Levels	Type of validation	Comments
❏ Experienced ❏ Need practice ❏ Never done ❏ Not applicable (based on scope of practice)	❏ Verbal ❏ Demonstration/ observation ❏ Practical exercise ❏ Interactive class	❏ Beginner ❏ Intermediate ❏ Expert	❏ Orientation ❏ Annual ❏ Other _____	

Employee signature

Observer signature

Name: ______________________________ Date: ______________

Skill: **Nursing Student Technician Competency Checklist**

Steps	Completed	Comments
A. Skills		
1. Basic care (bath, hair, teeth, ADLs).		
2. Ambulation.		
3. K-Pads.		
4. Ice bags.		
5. I & O documentation.		
6. Meal trays (administer & feed).		
7. Care of patient: a. With oxygen b. Stable postoperative c. With cast/splints (stable)		
8. Vital signs (BP, T, P, R).		
9. Obtain specimens a. Sputum b. Urine c. Stool		
10 Catheter care a. External male cath application b. Cath care		
11. Patient discharge (gather belongings & transfer).		
12. Team (CPR certification) a. Role in Team I b. dDefibrillation location (STH only)		
13. Morgue care (assist with care, transport body).		
14. Observational skills (reports s/s to RN).		
15. Transport patients, body mechanisms, and transfer techniques.		
16. Transfer patients.		
17. Valuables procedure.		
18. Weights: a. Bedside b. Portable		

19. Documentation a. Graphics sheet b. Dietary intake c. I&O d. IPN		
20. Enema.		
21. Catheterization a. Straight b. Foley		
22. Sterile/nonsterile compress.		
23. Skin preps.		
24. Traction.		
25. Dressing changes.		
26. Trach care.		
27. Suctioning.		
28. Blood draws (Note: No blood draws from central lines or PICCs)		

Self-assessment	Evaluation/ validation methods	Levels	Type of validation	Comments
❑ Experienced ❑ Need practice ❑ Never done ❑ Not applicable (based on scope of practice)	❑ Verbal ❑ Demonstration/ observation ❑ Practical exercise ❑ Interactive class	❑ Beginner ❑ Intermediate ❑ Expert	❑ Orientation ❑ Annual ❑ Other _____	

Employee signature

Observer signature

Name: ______________________________ Date: ______________

Skill: **Private Duty RN/LPN Competency Evaluation**

Steps	Completed	Comments
1. Demonstrates professional appearance, behavior, and confidentiality.		
2. Follows established policies and procedures within Summa Health System.		
3. Maintains patient safety through knowledge of emergency codes and appropriate actions (i.e., evaluation maps/safe areas).		
4. Verbalize the location of emergency equipment and the knowledge of C.P.R. procedure.		
5. Communicates appropriately with patient, family, and staff.		
6. Reports to the Registered Nurse/Designee prior to leaving patient unattended and upon returning to the unit from breaks.		
7. Implements body Substance Isolation precautions.		
8. Documents accurate implementation and evaluation of patient care.		
9. Follows through with proper IV maintenance by documenting and reporting all elements of IV therapy. **(RN Only)**.		
10. Administers, documents, and evaluates all medications appropriately according to Summa Health System policies and procedures. **(RN Only)**.		

Self-assessment	Evaluation/ validation methods	Levels	Type of validation	Comments
❑ Experienced ❑ Need practice ❑ Never done ❑ Not applicable (based on scope of practice)	❑ Verbal ❑ Demonstration/ observation ❑ Practical exercise ❑ Interactive class	❑ Beginner ❑ Intermediate ❑ Expert	❑ Orientation ❑ Annual ❑ Other _____	

Employee signature *Observer signature*

Name: ______________________________ Date: ______________

Skill: **Registration**

Steps	Completed	Comments
1. Greets patient/informs of need to gather information in manner consistent with house rules.		
2. Determines if patient has been previously registered within system; verifies birth date and Social Security number. If not previously registered, demonstrates knowledge registering new patient.		
3. Uses correct CPI number, continues through registration screens, asks pertinent questions, enters data.		
4. Demonstrates knowledge of using insurance master; identifies MC/MED/commercial insurance HMO/PPO.		
5. Demonstrates knowledge of Medicare secondary payer questionnaire asking patient-appropriate questions.		
6. Informs/requests patient to sign appropriate consent forms (i.e., surgical procedure, laser).		
7. Closes interview/registration with "thank you."		

Self-assessment	Evaluation/ validation methods	Levels	Type of validation	Comments
❑ Experienced ❑ Need practice ❑ Never done ❑ Not applicable (based on scope of practice)	❑ Verbal ❑ Demonstration/ observation ❑ Practical exercise ❑ Interactive class	❑ Beginner ❑ Intermediate ❑ Expert	❑ Orientation ❑ Annual ❑ Other _____	

______________________________ ______________________________

Employee signature *Observer signature*

Name: ______________________ Date: ______________

Skill: **RN Skills Assessment/Evaluation**

Steps	Completed	Comments
I. Competency: A. Applies a systematic problem-solving approach in the implementation of nursing plans of care: 1. Uses nursing process to systematically assess, plan, implement, and evaluate nursing care.		
2. Provide/documents patient teaching/discharge planning.		
3. Involves patient/significant other in plan of care.		
4. Prioritizes nursing care for a group of patients.		
5. Initiates patient referrals as needed.		
6. Utilizes appropriate resources.		
B. Intravenous Therapy 1. Initiates intravenous.		
2. Monitors intravenous according to policy and procedure: a. Checks rate		
b. Assesses for signs and symptoms of complications		
c. Initiates PRN adapter		
3. Uses infusion pumps correctly: • PCA		
• Baxter		
4. Draws blood specimens: • Routine		
• Central line		
• Blood cultures		
5. Administers blood and blood components.		
6. Maintains central line/hyperalimentation.		
7. Applies/changes central line dressing.		
8. Administers IV medications (I.V.P.B. IV push).		
9. Documents administration of IV Therapy.		

10. Completes IV Therapy exam with a minimum score of 80%.		
C. Medication Administration 1. Describes usual dose, common side effects, compatibilities, action, and untoward reactions of medications.		
2. Administers medications a. I.M.		
b. SQ and Insulin.		
c. Calculations.		
d. Other.		
3. Documents administration of medications (MAR, controlled drugs, etc.).		
4. Identifies medication error reporting system.		
D. Treatment and Procedures 1. Inserts and maintains gastric feeding tubes.		
2. Inserts and maintains urinary catheters.		
3. Performs trach care and suctioning.		
4. Assesses patient safety including proper utilization of restraints.		
5. Completes tissue therapy self-learning packet.		
6. Provides and documents pre- and postop nursing care.		
7. Incorporates nursing measures to reduce and prevent the spread of infection in daily nursing care.		
8. Completes American Heart Association guidelines for BLS-C in CPR.		
9. Changes oxygen gauge and sets rate.		
10. Locates various items on the emergency cart.		
11. Identifies nursing responsibilities in emergency situations.		
12. Completes: a. Admission of a patient.		
b. Transfer of a patient.		
c. Discharge of a patient.		
13. Performs neurological checks when appropriate.		

14. Performs BGT.		
15. Other.		
II. Communication A. Documents on the following forms: Initial Interdisciplinary Assessment		
1. Graphic Record		
2. Interdisciplinary Progress Record		
3. Nursing Discharge/Patient Teaching		
4. Interdisciplinary Plan of Care		
5. Unusual Occurrence		
B. Transcribes physicians' orders.		
C. Takes verbal orders from physician.		
D. Uses correct lines of communication.		
E. Attends Computer Class.		
F. Gives prompt, accurate, and pertinent shift report.		
G. Interacts with patients significant others and health team members in positive manner.		
III. Accountability/Leadership A. Completes orientation statement of agreement.		
B. Delegates patient care to other personnel appropriately.		
C. Follows appropriate employee policies and procedures, i.e. call off, time off, LOA, etc.		
D. Conforms to dress code.		
E. Identifies role of the nurse in quality assurance.		
F. Maintains safe working environment.		
G. Contains costs through proper use of supplies and maintenance of equipment.		
IV. Other: A. Has completed Human Resource/Safety Orientation.		

Self-assessment	Evaluation/ validation methods	Levels	Type of validation	Comments
❏ Experienced ❏ Need practice ❏ Never done ❏ Not applicable (based on scope of practice)	❏ Verbal ❏ Demonstration/ observation ❏ Practical exercise ❏ Interactive class	❏ Beginner ❏ Intermediate ❏ Expert	❏ Orientation ❏ Annual ❏ Other _____	

______________________________ ______________________________

Employee signature *Observer signature*

Name: ______________________ Date: ______________

Skill: **Sitter Guidelines/Expectations**

Steps	Completed	Comments
1. General Guidelines/Expectations Verbalizes or demonstrates: • Proper attire worn. • TV's and radios in patient's room are for the sole use of patient and not to be used by Float SA/Sitter Staff. • Food and beverages are not to be consumed in the patient's rooms.		
2. Lunches/Breaks/End of Shift Verbalizes or demonstrates: • Two (2) 15-minutes breaks and one half hour lunch during their 8-hour shift. • Break discussed with the RN responsible for the patient prior to starting their assignment. • Relief personnel present in the room before leaving for a break or lunch. • Use the call light to summon the nurse and ask for relief. If no relief at approved break and lunch. • **PATIENT NEVER LEFT ALONE UNTIL RELIEF PERSONNEL ARE AVAILABLE.** • Emergency requires sitter to leave the room at other than the scheduled break times, or if the next shift's sitter has not arrived by the end of your shift, summon the nurse, using the call light, to advise them that you need to leave the room. • Returning from lunch or break, reports to the Nursing Station to let them know of return.		

3. Patient Care Guidelines Verbalizes or demonstrates: • **DO NOT LEAVE THE PATIENT ATTENDED.** • Family visiting and asks sitter to leave the room. Stay in the immediate area of the patient's room so that you are aware of when the family leaves. A chair can be placed in the hall by the door to sit in while the family is visiting. • **DOES NOT SLEEP WHILE ON DUTY.** • Remain by the patient's bedside to assist them when taking fluids and nourishment, if permitted or directed, and to protect the patient from injury. • Does not comment or discuss patient or the family/visitors issues related to the patient's care, conditions or concerns about the nursing staff. • Alter to any change in the patient's behavior or condition (such as their breathing pattern, vomiting, restlessness, perspiring, pain or other signs or symptoms of difficulty and report these to unit personnel immediately. **Uses the call light to summon unit personnel immediately.**		
4. Patient Care Responsibilities Verbalized or demonstrates: • Assists the unit staff to change the bed linens and patient's gown if necessary. • Provides assistant to the unit staff with patient's shower or bath. • Assists patient with personal hygiene such as brushing their teeth, washing face and hands, etc. • Assists unit staff to turn patient when requested. • Under the direction of the nursing staff, assists the patient into a chair or to the bathroom. Float SA/Sitter is to remain with patient and assist them back to bed. • Intervenes to prevent patient from falling and pulling at tubes. If a patient falls, if it becomes difficult to keep patient from pulling their IV or tubes, or if it appears that a tube has been pulled out of place **UNIT STAFF SUMMONED IMMEDIATELY.** • Assists the patient with the bedpan or urinal as necessary. Measure urine output and report to the Nurse if so directed.		

5. Patient with Suicide Precautions Verbalized or demonstrates: • Restricts patient to his/her own room. Patient should not leave the room without constant staff accompaniment (i.e., diagnostic tests, treatments). **Accompany the patient off the unit. At no time is the patient to be out of your or another staff member's vision.** • Patient wears a hospital gown at all times. • Removes potentially hazardous items from the patient's environment. This includes, but is not limited to: alcoholic beverages, cleaning solutions, crochet hooks, electrical appliances, glass items, glass vases, hangers, knitting needles, knives, lighters, lotions, matches, medications, metal eating utensils, nail polish remover, needles/sharps containers, perfume, picture frames, pins, plastic bags, pop cans, razor blades, scissors, spray containers, thumb tacks, tweezers. • Surveys the environment for any restricted items. • **Restricted items may be used <u>ONLY</u> in the presence of a staff member.** • Reminds visitors not to leave potentially harmful items with the patient. • **Patients are not to be out of the sitter's vision when visitors are present.** • Patient belongings placed in a bag, labeled, and either sent home with the family or kept at nurse's station until patient's discharge. • Meal Tray Precautions: a. **Paper tray set-up** through dietary. b. When serves a patient, assure that paper cups and plates and plastic utensils are on the tray both before and after meals. Cuts food and remove the knife and fork. Finger foods OK. c. Reports any missing items to the Registered Nurse. • Patients are not permitted to wander in the hall. Report patient leaving room to RN. Don't lose sight of the patient. • Patients are not permitted to leave the unit AMA.		

Self-assessment	Evaluation/ validation methods	Levels	Type of validation	Comments
❑ Experienced ❑ Need practice ❑ Never done ❑ Not applicable (based on scope of practice)	❑ Verbal ❑ Demonstration/ observation ❑ Practical exercise ❑ Interactive class	❑ Beginner ❑ Intermediate ❑ Expert	❑ Orientation ❑ Annual ❑ Other _____	

Employee signature

Observer signature

Name: ______________________________ Date: ______________

Skill: **Telephone Skills**

Steps	Completed	Comments
1. Answers the telephone in three rings or less.		
2. Identifies self by department, title, and name in appropriate professional business tone and language.		
3. Asks caller how one can be of service (example: "How may I help you today?").		
4. Demonstrates placing caller on hold, checking back every 30 seconds or less while looking for additional information for the caller.		
5. Demonstrates transferring a call when the caller has accessed one's department incorrectly.		
6. Demonstrates taking a message: records caller's name, nature of message, telephone number, etc.		
7. Closes conversation with offers of any other assistance and thank you.		

Self-assessment	Evaluation/ validation methods	Levels	Type of validation	Comments
❑ Experienced ❑ Need practice ❑ Never done ❑ Not applicable (based on scope of practice)	❑ Verbal ❑ Demonstration/ observation ❑ Practical exercise ❑ Interactive class	❑ Beginner ❑ Intermediate ❑ Expert	❑ Orientation ❑ Annual ❑ Other _____	

______________________________ ______________________________

Employee signature *Observer signature*

Name: ______________________________ Date: ______________

Skill: **Telephone Skills (Problem Solving)**

Steps	Completed	Comments
1. Answers routine telephone calls by the third ring in a friendly manner by identifying his or her name and department.		
2. Refers to interdepartmental phone book and class schedules to help locate any employees or meetings in our buildings. Asks for clarification.		
3. Utilizes other staff members for telephone coverage while away from the desk area/has someone sit at the reception desk to cover the phone calls.		
4. Before leaving for lunch or break, asks who is available to cover the phone. Gives a time reference as to when he or she is leaving and will be returning.		
5. Notifies person when he or she returns.		
6. Keeps Rolodex up-to-date.		
7. Retrieves voicemail message in a timely manner and responds/follows through accordingly.		

Self-assessment	Evaluation/ validation methods	Levels	Type of validation	Comments
❑ Experienced ❑ Need practice ❑ Never done ❑ Not applicable (based on scope of practice)	❑ Verbal ❑ Demonstration/ observation ❑ Practical exercise ❑ Interactive class	❑ Beginner ❑ Intermediate ❑ Expert	❑ Orientation ❑ Annual ❑ Other _____	

______________________________ ______________________________

Employee signature *Observer signature*

Name: ______________________ Date: ______________

Skill: **Unit Secretary Orientation Skills Assessment/Evaluation**

Steps	Completed	Comments
I. Clinical Duties A. Transcription 1. Correctly identifies and transcribes/processes stat or other priority orders into PLATO.		
2. Correctly transcribes current medication orders onto the Medication Administration Record (MAR): • Processes orders from paper to PLATO. • Sends Home Medication List & Order sheet to Pharmacy if needed.		
3. Correctly transcribes Lab orders by: a. Completing requisitions, if needed.		
b. Notifying Nursing, and printing lab labels, placing in biohazard bag.		
c. Processing in PLATO, creating ADT logs, or other lists as unit appropriate.		
4. Correctly transcribes other Diagnostic orders and other physician consultations. a. (Radiology, Cardiology, Neurology Testing, etc.) • Completing Diagnostic Requisitions.		
b. Scheduling the diagnostic studies. 1) Calling physician office and/or 2) Clinical diagnostic test unit.		
c. Adding consulting physician to the patient provider list PLATO.		
d. Sending Notification of Added Physician message in (PLATO).		
e. Printing the appropriate Prep slips.		
5. Correctly transcribes Respiratory orders by accurately: a. Notifying Respiratory Therapy.		
b. Recording order on PLATO.		
6. Correctly transcribes Dietary orders by: a. Recording the order on the Diet Roster.		

b. Notifying Dietary of late orders.		
7. Correctly transcribes treatment orders by accurately: a. Entering order to PLATO.		
b. Notifying the department or technician of the order per flow-sheet procedure, if not automatically done in PLATO (i.e., Nutrition Support, RT or EKG).		
c. Ordering the appropriate patient care equipment.		
B. Manages patient chart assembly as required. 1. Admission		
2. Discharge		
3. Transfer • Sends PLATO message (Registration). • Notifies RN to create a current list of orders to be used on receiving unit (non-PLATO to PLATO).		
4. Pre/PostOp • Checklist review. • Generates patient information sheets, if available.		
5. Thinning charts (to "older" sections on unit). • Correctly removes only what is allowed to be thinned. • Recollates charts into one medical record at discharge.		
C. Notifies Patient Registration of Admissions, discharges, deaths, transfers or change of status. • Using Status Change Form. • Using PLATO system, when available.		
D. Completes chart rounds including: 1. Checks charts adding additional forms.		
2. Assures correct chart order.		
3. Places MAR's, reports or transfer record, etc., on chart in correct location.		
E. Sorts incoming mail/faxes and files in appropriate charts.		
F. Uses and files OR, Radiology, PT or other schedules as appropriate resources.		

G. Completes and updates, as appropriate: 1. Supervisor's Report or Optilink™ review.		
2. Dietary Roster, sending messages to Dietary or phoning with updated information.		
3. Daily Work List (i.e., form 90200150) if used.		
4. ADT Loq.		
5. Consult Log.		
6. Communication Board.		
7. Bulletin Boards.		
8. Routine Labs (serial and daily).		
9. Census Check in OptiLink™.		
10. Central Transport list of transfers.		
11. Shift Flags turned on and off in PLATO.		
12. **Other unit-based competencies as required.**		
H. Demonstrate Use of 1. Telephone (Desk and Electronic)		
2. Patient Intercom		
3. Page System		
4. Pneumatic Tube		
5. Lab Label Printer & Addressograph imprinter		
6. Copy Machine		
7. Care Windows Class/PLATO Class		
8. Central Transport In-Patient Request call Notification of Transfer (to unit or morgue) • Enters Medical Record # without extra 00s		
9. E-mail class		
10. Fax Machine		
• Adding paper		
• Adding toner		
II. Clerical Duties A. Orders office supplies as needed.		
B. Orders forms as needed.		
III. Examination Completes the Medical Terminology exam with a minimum score of 80%.		
IV. Basic Lift Support (Circle One) **HeartSaver CPR** **Health Care Provider**		

V. Communication		
1. Reads email and prints communication to staff / places on unit bulletin board as needed.		
2. Sends pager text message and receives feedback from person paged.		
3. Documents a page returned on Consult Lob.		
VI. Human Relations A. Gives prompt, accurate, shift report to on-coming unit secretary		
B. Arrives on time in uniform.		
C. Notifies Nursing Administration Office and unit of absenteeism according to policy.		
D. Notifies unit manager and nursing administration office of tardiness according to policy.		
E. Notifies nurse in charge when leaving unit consistently.		
F. Follows current guidelines for breaks and lunch.		
G. Emails Staff Development Instructor with preceptor's name.		
VIII. Personal Appearance A. Conforms to dress code.		
IX. Completes self-learning packets as appropriate:		
New Employee Orientation		
MOE: • Fire/Electrical Safety • Evacuation • Hazard Communication • Infection Control • Weather Emergencies • Codes: Adam, Black, Blue, Red, Violet, Yellow		
X. Knows Armband colors • High Risk Falls armband alert • Allergy • Admission		

Self-assessment	Evaluation/ validation methods	Levels	Type of validation	Comments
❑ Experienced ❑ Need practice ❑ Never done ❑ Not applicable (based on scope of practice)	❑ Verbal ❑ Demonstration/ observation ❑ Practical exercise ❑ Interactive class	❑ Beginner ❑ Intermediate ❑ Expert	❑ Orientation ❑ Annual ❑ Other _____	

_______________________________ _______________________________

Employee signature *Observer signature*

Bibliography

General

Alvare, S., Dugan, D., and Fuzy, J. 2005. *Nursing Assistant Care.* Albuquerque, NM: Hartman Publishing.

American College of Cardiology and the American Heart Association 2004. ACC/AHA *Guideline for the Management of Patients With ST-Elevation Myocardial Infarction Pocket Guide.*

American Geriatrics Society, British Geriatrics Society, and American Academy of Orthopaedic Surgeons Panel on Falls Prevention. 2001. Guidelines for the prevention of falls in older persons. *Journal of the American Geriatrics Society* 49(5): 664-672.

American Heart Association. 2005. American Heart Association guidelines for cardiopulmonary resuscitation and emergency cardiovascular care. *Circulation* 112: IV35-IV46.

Brunt, B. 2007. *Competencies for Staff Educators: Tools to Evaluate and Enhance Nursing Professional Development.* Marblehead, MA: HCPro, Inc.

Doloresco, L., Lloyd, T., Smith, L., and Weinel, D. 2002. A clinical evaluation of ceiling lifts: Lifting and transfer technology for the future. *SCI Nurse* 19(2): 75-77.

Duell, D., Martin, B., and Smith, S. 2008. *Clinical Nursing Skills: Basic to Advanced Skills.* 7th ed. Upper Saddle River, NJ: Pearson Education, Inc.

Gazmuri, R. et al. 2007. Scientific knowledge gaps and clinical research priorities for cardiopulmonary resuscitation and emergency cardiac care identified during the 2005 international consensus conference on E and CPR science with treatment recommendations: A consensus statement from the International Liaison Committee on Resuscitation, the American Heart Association Emergency Cardiovascular Care Committee, the Stroke Council and Cardiovascular Nursing Council. *Circulation* 116: 2501-2512.

National Heart Lung and Blood Institute. 2007. *Deep Vein Thrombosis.* United States Department of Health and Human Services.

Nissen, S., Pepine, C., Bashore, T., et al. 1994. American College of Cardiology position statement. Cardiac angiography without cine film: erecting a "tower of Babel" in the cardiac catheterization laboratory. *Journal of the American College of Cardiology* 24: 834-837.

Perry, A. and Potter, P. 2006. *Clinical Nursing Skills & Techniques.* 6th Ed. St. Louis, MO: Mosby.

Studer, Q. 2003. *Hardwiring Excellence.* Gulf Breeze, FL: Fire Starter Publishing.

United States Department of Labor Occupational Safety and Health Administration. Fit testing guidelines. Standards 29CFR 1910.134, Appendix A.

Urdern, L., Stacy, K., and Lough, M., eds. 2006. *Thelan's Critical Care Nursing: Diagnosis and Management.* 5th ed. St. Louis, MO: Mosby Elsevier.

Weinstein, S. 2007. *Plumer's Principles and Practice of Intravenous Therapy. 8th ed.* Philadelphia, PA: Lippincott.

Intensive Care Unit

Aehlert, B. 2006. *Pocket Reference for ECGs Made Easy.* 3rd ed. St. Louis, MO: Mosby Elsevier.

Alspach, J. 2006. *Core Curriculum for Critical Care Nursing.* 6th ed. Saunders.

American College of Cardiology and the American Heart Association. 2004. *ACC/AHA Guideline for the Management of Patients With ST-Elevation Myocardial Infarction Pocket Guide.*

American Heart Association. 2005. Guidelines for cardiopulmonary resuscitation and emergency cardiovascular care. *Circulation* 112(Supp. 24): IV1-IV211.

Barker, E. 2002. *Neuroscience Nursing: A Spectrum of Care.* 2nd ed. Philadelphia, PA: Mosby.

Barthel, D., and Mahoney, F. 1965. Functional evaluation: the Barthel Index. *Maryland State Medical Journal* 14: 56-61.

Bell-Syer, S., et al. 2004. Support surfaces for pressure ulcer prevention. *Cochrane Database of Systematic Reviews* 3: CD001735.

Berenholtz, S, Milanovich, S, et al. 2004. Improving care for the ventilated patient. *Journal of Quality and Safety* 30(4): 195-204.

Calabrese, D. and Modic, M. "Renal and Urologic Care"in *Nursing Procedures.* 3rd ed. Springhouse, PA: Springhouse Corporation. 595-597.

Carlson, K. and Weigand, D. 2005. *AACN Procedure Manual for Critical Care.* 5th ed. St. Louis, MO: Elsevier Saunders.

Cheitlin, M., et al. 2003. ACC/AHA/ASE 2003 guideline update for the clinical application of echocardiography. *Journal of the American College of Cardiology* September 3, 2003.

Crawford, M. and Drake, J. 2005. Near miss injection of an anesthetic agent into a cerebrospinal fluid external ventricular drain: Special report. *Neurosurgery* 56(5): E116.

Crunden, E., Boyce, C., et al. 2005. An evaluation of the impact of the ventilator care bundle. *Nursing Critical Care* 10(5): 242-246.

Del Monte, L., Gamrath, B., and Richards, K. Noninvasive pacing: What you should know. *Journal of Emergency Nursing* 24(3): 223-232.

Duell, D., Martin, B., and Smith, S. 2008. *Clinical Nursing Skills: Basic to Advanced Skills.* 7th ed. Upper Saddle River, NJ: Pearson Education, Inc.

Fields, L., Blackshear, C., et al. 2005. *Guide to the Patient with Intracranial Pressure Monitoring: AACN Reference Series for Clinical Practice.* Chicago, IL: AACN.

Hill-Rom, Inc. 2005. Hill-Rom's new bariatric bed addresses growing obesity trend; designed to safely and comfortably support patients up to 1,000 pounds. *Obesity and Diabetes Week* July 4, 2005.

Hogg, M. and Kibbe, M. 2006. Percutaneous thoracic and abdominal aortic aneurysm repair: techniques outcomes. *Vascular* 14(5): 270-281.

Huijbregts, H. et al. 2008. Hemodialysis arteriovenous fistula patency revisited: Results of a prospective, multicenter initiative. *Clinical Journal of the American Society of Nephrology* February 2008.

Lough, M., Stacy, K., and Urden, L. 2006. Thelan's Critical Care Nursing: *Diagnosis and Management.* 5th ed. St Louis, MO: Mosby Elsevier.

Perry, A. and Potter, P. 2006. *Clinical Nursing Skills & Techniques.* 6th ed. St. Louis, MO: Mosby Elsevier.

Nursing education instructional guide

Target audience:

- Chief nursing officer
- Chief nurse executive
- Directors of nursing
- Directors of nursing education
- VPs of nursing
- Nurse managers
- Staff educators
- Staff development specialist
- Human resource professional

Statement of need:

Organizations have to conduct regular staff competency assessments, and fulfilling Joint Commission competency requirements are a key part of the staff education role. As evidence-based practice has become the norm for nursing, educators are looking for competency assessments that are based on evidence. The second edition of this book ensures competencies are based on best evidence.

Educational objectives:

Upon completion of this activity, participants should be able to:

- Design a competency plan to effectively assess employee competence
- Identify advantages of competency-based education
- Describe methods of validating competencies
- Recognize the benefits of incorporating competency assessment into job descriptions and performance evaluation tools

- Discuss the key elements required of performance-based job descriptions
- Develop a training program to train staff to perform competency assessment
- Maintain consistency in a competency validation system
- Identify steps for effective program documentation
- Recognize the essential qualities needed by competency assessors
- List potential categories for new competencies
- Identify best practices for implementing new competencies
- Discuss dimensions of competencies
- Differentiate between orientation checklists and skill checklists

Faculty:

Barbara A. Brunt, MA, MN, RN-BC

Adrianne E. Avillion, DEd, RN

Gwen A. Valois, MS, RN, BC

Jane G. Alberico, MS, RN, CEN

Accreditation/designation statement:

This educational activity for three contact hours is provided by HCPro, Inc. HCPro, Inc. is accredited as a provider of continuing nursing education by the American Nurses Credentialing Center's Commission on Accreditation.

Disclosure statements:

Barbara A. Brunt, Adrianne E. Avillion, Gwen A. Valois, and Jane G. Alberico have declared that they have no commercial/financial vested interest in this activity.

Instructions:

In order to be eligible to receive your nursing contact hour(s) for this activity, you are required to do the following:

1. Read the book
2. Complete the exam
3. Complete the evaluation
4. Provide your contact information in the space provided on the exam and evaluation
5. Submit the exam and evaluation to HCPro, Inc.

Please provide all of the information requested above and mail or fax your completed exam, program evaluation, and contact information to:

HCPro, Inc.
ATTN: Continuing Education Department
200 Hoods Lane
Marblehead, MA 01945
Tel: 877/727-1728
Fax: 781/639-2982

Nursing education exam

Name: ____

Title: ____

Facility name: ____

Address: ____

Address: ____

City: ______________________ State: ______________ ZIP: ________

Phone number: ______________________ Fax number: ______________________

E-mail: ____

Nursing license number: ____

(ANCC requires a unique identifier for each learner)

1. When designing a competency plan, attention must be paid to all of the following except:

   a. The needs of the patients and families

   b. The extended community

   c. Former standards of practice

   d. Organizational policies and procedures

2. "Competent" can be defined as:

   a. Well-qualified, capable, fit

   b. Underqualified, weak

   c. Underachieving

   d. Levelheaded

3. Which of the following is not a benefit of a competency-based approach?

   a. Reducing staff anxiety

   b. Increasing staff retention

   c. Encouraging independence instead of teamwork

   d. Enhancing skills and knowledge

4. Competency involves what domains of practice?

    a. Cognitive, affective, and psychomotor

    b. Cognitive, disaffective, and psychomotor

    c. Cognitive, affective, and psychosomatic

    d. Intuitive, affective, and psychosomatic

5. All of the following are methods for validating competency except:

    a. Posttests

    b. Case studies

    c. Simulated events

    d. Estimations

6. Observations of daily work to ensure competency can include:

    a. Patient rounds

    b. Phone calls

    c. Staff conversations

    d. Family discussions

7. Which of the following is not a benefit of incorporating competency assessment into job descriptions and performance evaluation tools?

    a. Improved efficiency

    b. Improved patient safety

    c. Improved employee satisfaction

    d. Improved nurse/physician communication

8. Practice standards in a well-developed competency- or performance-based job description should be:
   a. Subjective
   b. Measurable and objective
   c. Vague to interpretation
   d. Age-specific

9. When incorporating competency-based performance standards in job descriptions, sections should be devoted to all of the following except:
   a. Teamwork
   b. Mandatory safety requirements
   c. Communication
   d. Independence

10. Which of the following is not a component of a competency assessment training and education program?
    a. Purpose
    b. Learning styles
    c. Maintaining objectivity
    d. Withholding criticism

11. All of the following are principles of adult learning except:
    a. Adults must have a valid reason for learning
    b. Adults do not bring life experiences to a learning situation
    c. Adults are self-directed learners
    d. Adults respond to both extrinsic and intrinsic motivators

12. Consistency in documentation:

   a. is as important as consistency in approach

   b. is not as important as consistency in approach

   c. does not relate to consistency in approach

   d. results in consistency in approach

13. All of the following are common job titles that may carry with them the responsibility for competency assessment except:

   a. Preceptor

   b. Nurse manager

   c. Staff development specialist

   d. Unit secretary

14. To keep your validation system consistent, you should always maintain ________.

   a. Subjectivity

   b. Objectivity

   c. Biases

   d. Partiality

15. Which of the following is not a qualification a competency assessor should possess?

   a. Mediocre performance of the competencies being evaluated

   b. The desire to acquire or enhance adult education skills

   c. Demonstration of excellent interpersonal communication skills

   d. Tact and the desire to help colleagues improve their job performance

16. What is not an essential component of competency documentation?

    a. Assessment documentation must be dated.

    b. Identify the specific competency being assessed.

    c. Identify the objectives that must be achieved to demonstrate competency.

    d. Document nonspecific steps in competency achievement.

17. All of the following are potential categories for new competencies except:

    a. New medications

    b. Old equipment

    c. Interpersonal communications

    d. New patient populations

18. What is not a best practice for implementing new competencies?

    a. Competency skills fairs

    b. Drills

    c. Self-assessment

    d. Word of mouth

19. The three dimensions of competencies include:

    a. Critical-thinking dimension, interpersonal dimension, and technical dimension

    b. Critical-thinking dimension, selective dimension, and scientific dimension

    c. Cognitive-thinking dimension, selective dimension, and technical dimension

    d. Correlated dimension, interpersonal dimension, and scientific dimension

20. The purpose of a competency program is to do all of the following except:

    a. Improve job performance

    b. Decrease organizational effectiveness

    c. Enhance patient outcomes

    d. Promote economic efficiency

21. Orientation checklists specify the ___, ____, and ____ needed to perform safely.

    a. techniques, abilities, and background

    b. intelligence, opinions, and viewpoints

    c. methods, talents, and capabilities

    d. knowledge, attitudes, and skills

22. Skills checklists should be:

    a. Learner oriented

    b. Unfocused on behaviors

    c. Ambiguous

    d. Immeasurable

Nursing education evaluation

Name: ______________________________

Title: ______________________________

Facility name: ______________________________

Address: ______________________________

Address: ______________________________

City: ____________________ State: ________ ZIP: ____________

Phone number: ______________ Fax number: ______________

E-mail: ______________________________

Nursing license number: ______________________________

(ANCC requires a unique identifier for each learner)

1. This activity met the following learning objectives:

a.) Designed a competency plan to effectively assess employee competence

Strongly disagree 1 2 3 4 5 Strongly agree

b.) Identified advantages of competency-based education

Strongly disagree 1 2 3 4 5 Strongly agree

c.) Determined methods of validating competencies

Strongly disagree 1 2 3 4 5 Strongly agree

d.) Recognized the benefits of incorporating competency assessment into job descriptions and performance evaluation tools

Strongly disagree 1 2 3 4 5 Strongly agree

e.) Discussed the key elements required of performance-based job descriptions

Strongly disagree 1 2 3 4 5 Strongly agree

f.) Developed a training program to train staff to perform competency assessment

Strongly disagree 1 2 3 4 5 Strongly agree

g.) Maintained consistency in a competency validation system

Strongly disagree 1 2 3 4 5 Strongly agree

h.) Identified steps for effective program documentation

Strongly disagree 1 2 3 4 5 Strongly agree

i.) Recognized the essential qualities needed by competency assessors

Strongly disagree 1 2 3 4 5 Strongly agree

j.) Listed potential categories for new competencies

Strongly disagree 1 2 3 4 5 Strongly agree

k.) Identified best practices for implementing new competencies

Strongly disagree 1 2 3 4 5 Strongly agree

l.) Discussed dimensions of competencies

Strongly disagree 1 2 3 4 5 Strongly agree

m.) Differentiated between orientation checklists and skill checklists

Strongly disagree 1 2 3 4 5 Strongly agree

2. Objectives were related to the overall purpose/goal of the activity.

Strongly disagree 1 2 3 4 5 Strongly agree

3. This activity was related to my nursing activity needs.

Strongly disagree 1 2 3 4 5 Strongly agree

4. The exam for the activity was an accurate test of the knowledge gained.

Strongly disagree 1 2 3 4 5 Strongly agree

5. The activity avoided commercial bias or influence.

Strongly disagree 1 2 3 4 5 Strongly agree

6. This activity met my expectations.

Strongly disagree 1 2 3 4 5 Strongly agree

7. Will this learning activity enhance your professional nursing practice?

Yes No

8. This educational method was an appropriate delivery tool for the nursing/clinical audience.

Strongly disagree 1 2 3 4 5 Strongly agree

9. How committed are you to making the behavioral changes suggested in this activity?

a. Very committed

b. Somewhat committed

c. Not committed

10. Please provide us with your degree.

a. ADN

b. BSN

c. MSN

d. Other, please state

11. Please provide us with your credentials.

a. LVN

b. LPN

c. RN

d. NP

e. Other, please state

12. Providing nursing contact hours for this product influenced my decision to buy it.

Strongly disagree 1 2 3 4 5 Strongly agree

13. I found the process to obtain my continuing education credits for this activity easy to complete.

Strongly disagree 1 2 3 4 5 Strongly agree

14. If you did not find the process easy to complete, which of the following areas did you find the most difficult?

a. Understanding the content of the activity

b. Understanding the instructions

c. Completing the exam

d. Completing the evaluation

e. Other, please state:

15. How much time did it take for you to complete this activity (this includes reading the book and completing the exam and the evaluation)? ____________________

____

16. If you have any comments on this activity, process, or selection of topics for nursing CE, please note them below.

____

____

____

____

17. Would you be interested in participating as a pilot tester for the development of future HCPro nursing education activities?

Yes No

Thank you for completing this evaluation of our nursing CE activity!